The Rider *forms* the Horse

Function and Development of
the Muscles of the Riding Horse

Udo Bürger
&
Otto Zietzschmann

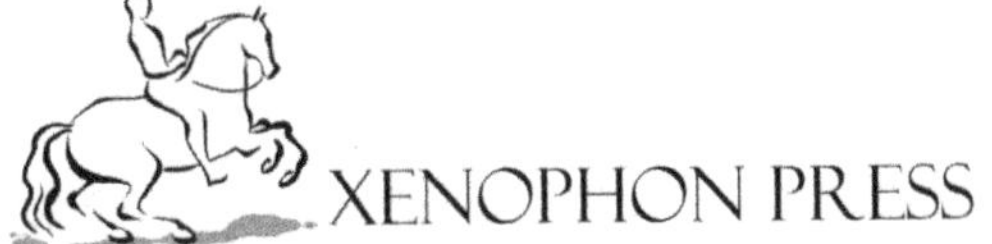

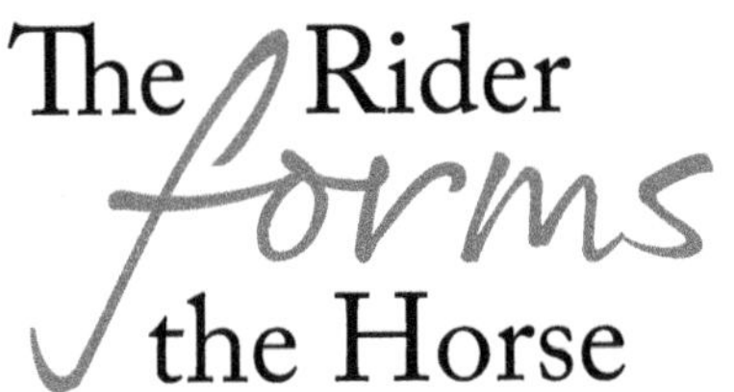

The Rider forms the Horse

Function and Development of
the Muscles of the Riding Horse

Dr. Udo Bürger
Veterinary Officer (with the equivalent rank of Major) and Chief Veterinary Officer
of the Cavalry Riding and Driving School Hanover

Dr. Dr. h. c. Otto Zietzschmann
Professor of anatomy at the School of Veterinary Medicine Hanover

This book is a reprint of the first edition which appeared in Germany in 1939. The photographs have been retained in their authentic form to maintain the integrity of the original book as they relate very closely to the text and only serve to better illustrate the training of the horse to the reader.
XENOPHON PRESS and **FN***verlag* do not identify with the uniforms and any possible ideological associations!

XENOPHON PRESS LLC
Franktown Virginia

German Edition:
National German Library bibliographical information:The National German Library lists this publication in the German National Bibliography; detailed bibliographic data is available on the internet at http://dnb.dnb.de.

First published in 1939 by Verlag M. & H. Scharper, Hanover

Publisher:
Deutsche Reiterliche Vereinigung e.V.; National Federation for Equestrian Sports and Breeding; Fédération Équestre Nationale (FN), Warendorf
FNVerlag German Edition ISBN 9783885426875

Illustrations:
The Anatomical Institute, School of Veterinary Medicine, Hanover

Cover: Thiedemann; Sportfotos Stefan Lafrentz, Plön

Photographs: Tiedemann (14 pictures); Wisskirchen (1 picture); Private (3 pictures)
Film: Heeresbildstelle (Army photographic office), Berlin; Werner Ernst, Ganderkesee: Pages 15, 16
Menzendorf, item on loan by the Sparkassenstiftung Lower-Saxony and the Kreissparkasse Verden at the German Horse Museum, Verden/Aller: pages 13, 14; Arnd Bronkhorst Horse Photography, Garderen/NL: page 19; Fotohaus Kiepker, Lengerich: page 17; Roger Muller/ROM Photography, Donaueschingen: page 19; Guido Recki, Dorsten: page 18

Layout and cover design:
Katja van Ravenstein, www.ravenstein2.de

New Xenophon Press Edition 2024
Translation: Teresa Hoffmann, Norwich/Norfolk, GBR
Revision 2021: Lena Rindermann, Warendorf, GER; Dr. Anastasios Moschos, Warendorf, GER
Design and layout by Robert Ashbaugh Digital Design and Imaging. Tucson, AZ
Cover Image: Westphalian mare, Frau Holle, ridden by Jana Schrödter at Donaueschingen 2020.

Requests for permission should be addressed to
Xenophon Press LLC,
7518 Bayside Road,
Franktown Virginia 23354-2106
email: XenophonPress@gmail.com

Xenophon Press English Edition ISBN: 9781948717564

Contents

Foreword

It is a great pleasure for me to be asked to write the foreword to this edition of *The Rider forms the Horse* by Udo Bürger and Otto Zietschmann. The book was out of print for several years and, in my opinion, it should be compulsory reading for all professionals or keen horse people who want to responsibly study the training of the horse. I would like to warmly thank all those at **FN***verlag*, and now Xenophon Press who have been responsible for bringing out this new edition of the book which first appeared in 1939.

Recently, one of the best-known horse breeders in Germany said to me: "The quality of horses has improved so much over the last few decades. Unfortunately, the training of the riders has not kept pace with breeding. Success is based 75% on training and 25% on the innate predisposition of the horse." From personal experience, I can only emphasize this statement. Untold numbers of "top horses" disappear, never to be seen again, as a result of incorrect training, whilst other difficult horses of rather average talent are formed into "top horses" by good trainers.

What is absolutely essential for the training of the horse is an understanding of the connections between muscular function and the skeleton and their interplay during the different phases of training and movements. This applies to whichever equestrian discipline has been chosen.

Dr. Udo Bürger was the chief veterinary officer at the famous "Cavalry School" in Hanover and Dr. h.c. Otto Zietzschmann was professor of anatomy at the School of Veterinary Medicine in Hanover. Both were active riders and in close contact with each other as well as with the world-class riders of the Cavalry School. They knew what they were talking about. In my opinion, they have left us a rare jewel in the form of this book.

The triumphs of German riding are founded on the sound all-round equine knowledge which was taught to an exemplary standard at the Cavalry School in Hanover. And the School was the right place to do so. They had "schoolmasters" in the very best meaning of the word, on which the unexperienced rider could "learn how it feels," when the back is swinging and the horse stretches trustingly toward the bit and into the rider's hands, when the hindquarters are engaged, or the horse reacts willingly to a half-halt. In those days, time was invested in training these horses, an investment which was advantageous for the long and healthy life of the horse and for the harmony between horse and rider. Exercising horses, and especially young horses, outside in the fresh air was natural, but even at an advanced stage of training, working in open countryside was an integral part of the schooling of the horses and riders training, as was riding over obstacles (for more on this subject see Chapter 12).

Plenty of staff were employed to care for all the horses' needs. All this has changed radically. Horses have become consumer goods which have to be sold as quickly as possible for the highest possible price. It is the breeders who usually profit the least from this development. Many trainers have never had the opportunity to experience the feel of a well-ridden horse and, very often, in-depth knowledge of equestrian facts as presented in this book is, unfortunately, lacking.

I have often asked myself in my role as a trainer, whether it is possible to re-educate the 'feeling' of riders on their horses – some of which are totally tense – and give them an idea of how it should really feel.

Riders often resort quickly to auxiliary aids as, for example, draw reins, to make their task easier. Unfortunately, this is the case even in well-known dressage facilities. Very few people realize that this is, in fact, incompetence on the part of the rider as well as abuse of the animal. Vets, chiropractors, osteopaths, and acupuncturists are then called in to treat the damages which have been caused. Auxiliary aids of every sort should be superfluous in correct training.

Personally, I was extremely fortunate to have had a trainer from the Hanover Cavalry School in the person of Otto Hartwich, commander of the mounted police squadron in Düsseldorf. He was an excellent rider and trainer, who adhered to all the rules of the classical school. He made me understand that basic work has to precede every movement. He taught me how it feels when the horse begins to dance under the rider and also when the horse's back is strong enough for the highest level of collection. He also taught me that the rider may accept collection even from young horses if they are not forced to do it, and that force makes both, the rider and the horse, tense and, therefore, can cause injuries. You could see how his horses became more beautiful during the course of training. He made me understand that competition success is not everything and that we have a duty toward the horses, which are entrusted to us and at our mercy at the same time.

I have re-discovered many of his thoughts in this book. Even today, I often pick up this book when a problem arises, which I have not previously experienced. Horses often confront even the experienced rider with new challenges and with the realization that nothing is totally predictable in this profession, and that a human life is not long enough to learn to ride. In the same spirit, I hope you enjoy reading this educational and interesting book.

Klaus Balkenhol – Olympic Champion and former German national trainer

Thoughts on the Book

Introductory Words

To find the right words to introduce a book which is just as contemporary now as when it was written back in 1939 is not at all easy. Nevertheless, dear reader, I shall attempt to do so, and to elucidate the special qualities of this brilliant book.

At the time this book was written, the equestrian sport was mostly confined to a certain social class and, simply for economic reasons, could only be engaged in by a small privileged social class. Horses were rather needed for use in war. They were trained in the military riding schools, the custodians of the doctrines of classical riding. These cavalry schools frequently produced older riding school horses which had been retired from military service and were much sought-after as schoolmasters by civilian riders. In those days, however, commercial aspects did not yet play a role in the training of horses.

It was not until the post-war years that the equestrian sport began to expand so extensively and people from all levels of society became involved in the training of horses. Nowadays, we differentiate between leisure or amateur and so-called professional equestrian sport. Our leisure-time riders are mostly highly motivated but frequently lack experience in handling horses as well as a basic understanding of the links and correlations in the equine body. This lack of knowledge results in many mistakes in training, which, ultimately, is detrimental to the horse, psychologically and also physically.

The professionals on the equestrian scene, however, usually have a sound fundamental knowledge. Nevertheless, many of them are not really familiar with the deeper connections. Besides, quite frequently, the commercial aspect is of such importance that fast-track training very often brings fast financial rewards – it is, however, not the way to long-lasting success.

Insufficient knowledge of anatomical and physiological connections reveals its greatest failings in the area of working with young horses in their 1st and 2nd years of training. The major sources of mistakes become apparent in the first years of basic training. Many riders believe that training a horse first and foremost means training to obey and carry out movements. In reality, however, this mechanical component plays a rather subordinate role. Furthermore, nowadays new ideas are quite suddenly propagated which encourage people to think that there could be other ways of attaining the desired goal.

This book, however, explains very clearly the importance of allowing a horse's body to develop. In other words, one could say that we accompany a process of development and change, which takes place over a period of months and years.

It is exactly this "time" factor which appears to no longer be available today. The long, slow path described in *The Rider forms the Horse*, which, generally, also does not lead to fast financial reward, promotes the health and robustness of horses. A great deal of detailed anatomical knowledge combines with established facts relating to the physiology of training and defines a way of training, which, aside from some minor individual variations, describes the common theme applied to the development of any young horse (remount). It becomes clearly recognizable that the factor of time, in conjunction with a certain level of technical ability on the part of the rider, and especially with the basic requirement of a calm, balanced, and contented rider, plays the greatest part in this responsible task of training the horse.

At the beginning of training, a bridge constructed for horizontal forward movement is suddenly subjected to a vertical load. Young horses are very fragile, easily injured, and weak. How do these bodies react to this different weight? At first – understandably – with defensive tension and stiffening. Only sufficient basic knowledge of natural behavioral patterns and physical interactions allow us to accustom the horse to the weight, to help it to overcome stiffening, and to let the actual training commence. The aim is to allow this young animal to develop in such a way that it will become a marvelous, light-footed, balanced, and healthy riding horse.

By now, dear readers, you will all be aware that the most important steps a horse must take along the path towards becoming a complete riding horse are at the very beginning. The principles of classical horsemanship and riding theory define a path which shows us how we can change this large muscular body without damaging or destroying it. In addition, it should be clear to everybody that a process of remodeling the body is accompanied by intense muscular pains.

If you take up a sport tomorrow which is completely new to you, you will find this an extremely demanding experience for you. How is it that so many people forget this experience which they have had in their own lives?

Why must so many horses continue to work in spite of extreme muscle pain and, ultimately, suffer because of the ignorance or lack of sensitivity of their riders? This reckless type of training does not give the rider any pleasure either. Furthermore, horses which have been ridden with artificially created tension lose their beauty, spirit, and harmony. They suffer tense back muscles in their moments of suspension and show a high knee action with their front limbs. These occasionally impressive show steps do not, however, require sufficient suppleness. Susceptibility to injuries increases considerably as a result. Repeated incidences of lameness affecting the joints is often an indication of such incorrect work. Insufficient suppleness, also in the region of the limbs, leads to an inadequate supply of nutrients to the joint cartilage with corresponding long-term repercussions in the joints. In the same way, regularly occurring soft tissue damage (tendon damage) indicates frequently working beyond the point of muscle exhaustion. One should never continue to exercise a horse when it is tired. Many of these elementary sport-associated physiological facts are unknown and unnecessarily lead to damage to the legs. In conjunction with all these physical problems, psychological damage often occurs in incorrectly and excessively exercised horses. But only a pain-free and supple body leads to a balanced inner self. Think about your mood, if you have acute back pains or a toothache. How keen are you then to work?

Many further questions will be answered in this book: How does a horse carry the rider's weight? How can it do this without being injured in the process? Naturally, such a large and powerful animal with its powerful muscles can bear a relatively heavy weight on its back! But how does it do this with light-footed elegance? How can a horse become more aesthetically pleasing, more beautiful, and more dynamic at the same time? A pack donkey bears its burden and wears itself out in the process. A correctly trained horse remains healthy, capable of high performances, and beautiful well into old age.

We will learn about the great importance of a well-developed head-neck-axis, which is as long as possible. We will be educated about what it means to shorten and tighten a young horse in the neck through dominant use of the hand. We will learn about the paramount importance of a supple swinging back for the whole course of training. We will also learn to use a giving rein aid. Riders who believes they can train a horse by the action of their hands will learn that they are on the wrong path, only leading to dissatisfaction. There are only few riders who have enough feeling to recognize situations where they should dismount or take their horse out for a walk hack. This book explains so much about horses and their development, and only with this knowledge will training a young horse be successful!

I wish you great pleasure and success with this book and your horse.

Dr. G. Heuschmann

Dr. Gerd Heuschmann – Warendorf March 2003/October 2021

A Message from the German Equestrian Federation (FN)

For the reasons that Dr. Heuschman so aptly points out, the **FN***verlag* has published a new series of re-edited, selected, and competent equestrian books – the "FN-Reprints." These give us an overview of the thoughts in equestrian sports in the 1930's. They portray an era in which the "modern riding" of today developed from its previous primarily military role into a civilian activity and competitive sport.

Dr. Udo Bürger was chief veterinary officer at the famous "Cavalry School" in Hanover and was in close contact with Dr. h.c. Otto Zietzschmann, professor of anatomy at the Veterinary School of Medicine in Hanover. Both were avid riders with close links to the world-class riders of the Cavalry School.

These reprints of equestrian masterpieces offer, without doubt, every reader the welcome opportunity to expand their knowledge of this field.

Heinz-Dieter Donner – held a management role in the areas of professional education, education of judges, and the development and compilation of teaching material at the German Equestrian Federation (FN) from 1974 to 1987.

Even Today,

the knowledge of the functional connections of the horse's anatomy remains of great importance for its training as a riding horse. The conflict between an age-appropriate physical development of the horse and the economic considerations of breeders, raisers, owners, trainers, and riders related to training young horses must, for the most part, be regulated through clear standards set by breeding and sport organizations. These rules can be adjusted when required. The explanation and objective derivation why an early, yet moderately developing training process over a longer period of time is vital for the horse, but still profitable for the owner or rider, can be found in this book, which remains significant to this day. Dr. Gerd Heuschmann kindly helped this book, dating back to 1939, to renewed attention at the beginning of the millennium, when he pointed out that there is no publication that explains these important connections in a better way. Hence, it is a very welcome initiative that the **FN***verlag* reprints this book once again

Thies Kaspareit – Head of the Education and Training Department at the German Equestrian Federation (FN)
Warendorf October 2021

The Development of Riding Horses

Herder

Shilfa xx
Perfectionist xx
Monsieur Gabriel xx
Pilger

Brown | Gelding | born 1931

Herdmütterchen
Parsee xx

Through the training of Herder, Felix Bürkner impressively documented for posterity the positive effect of classical equitation and manifested the soundness of the theses presented by Udo Bürger and Otto Zietzschmann in this book.

Herder as a young horse under Felix Bürkner

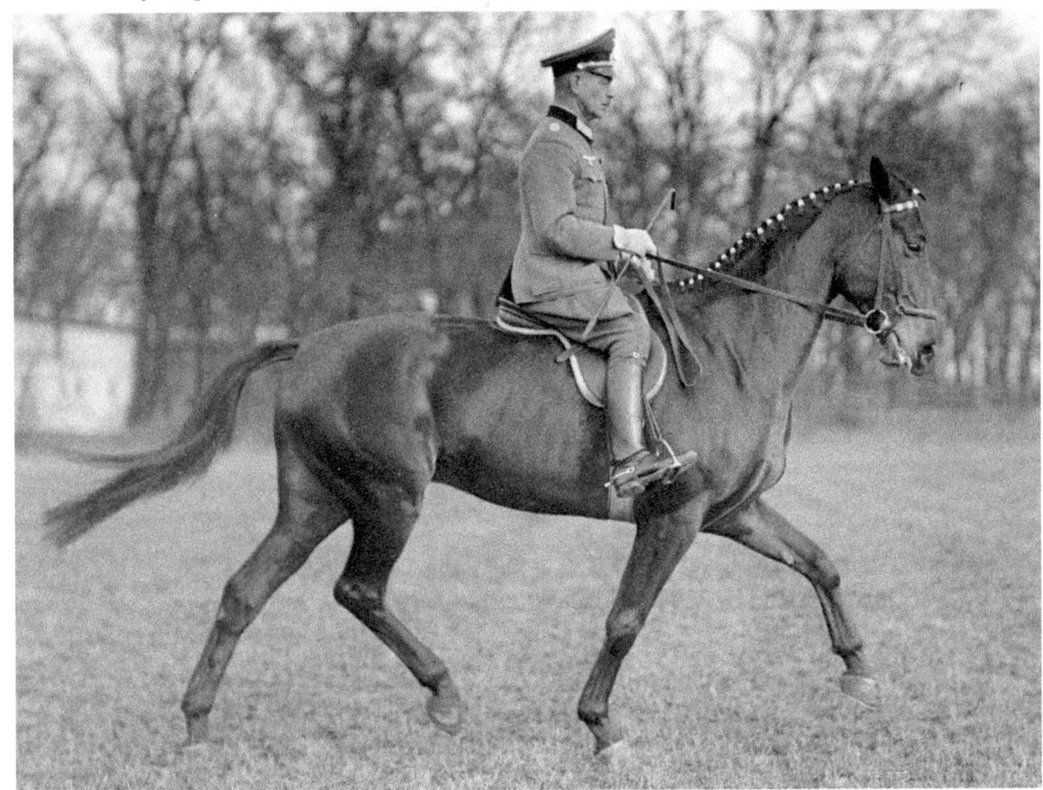

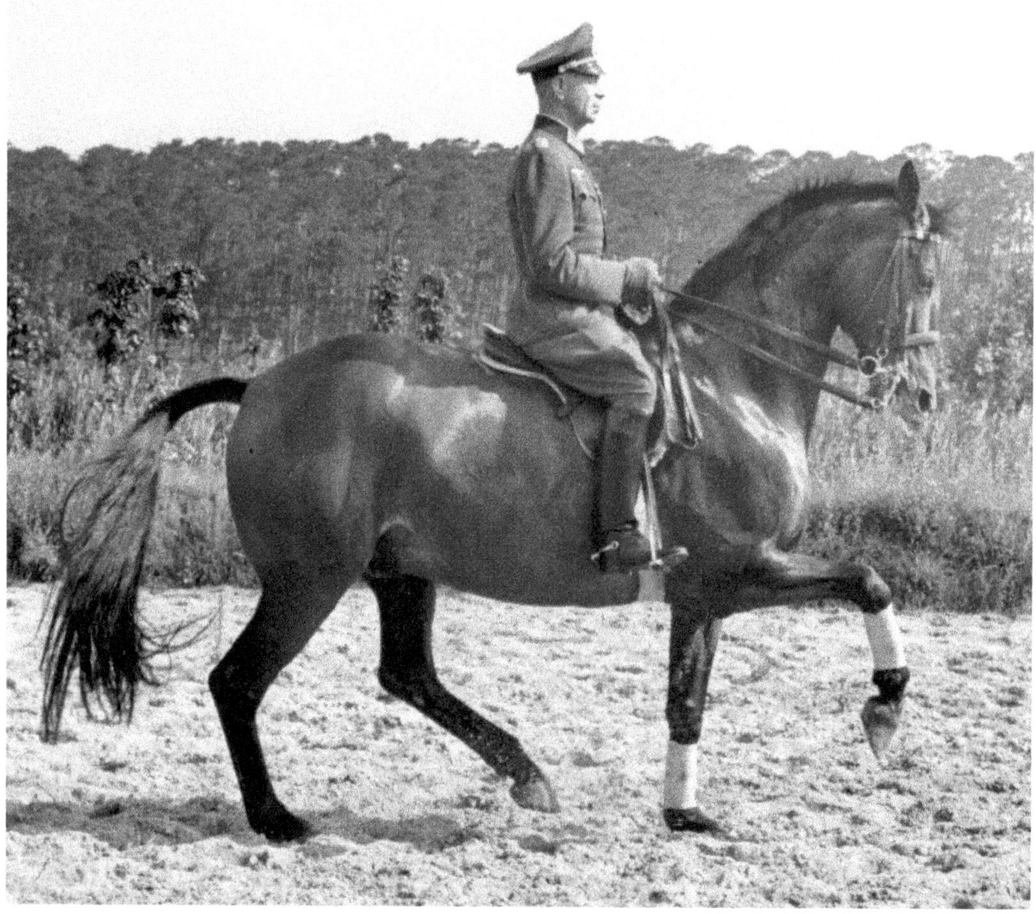

Herder under Felix Bürkner in the passage

The positive effect of the gymnasticizing process is demonstrated in impressive fashion by the example of the horse "Herder": At the beginning of his career in 1937 Herder shows little muscular development and is not yet balanced under his rider. Bürkner consistently rode this horse forward for a year without collection.

After 6 years of consistent work, Herder can hardly be recognized as the same horse. But it is! This shows how systematic training can change a horse. Bürkner rode Herder consistently from back to front – over the back, through the poll, and into the hand. The rider's forward driving aids always took priority over the regulating ones. The horse seeks the contact. The rider allows it.

Donnerhall

Disput
Donnerwetter
Melli

Chestnut | Stallion | born 1981

Markus
Ninette
Negola

Donnerhall was approved during the 1982 Oldenburg stallion licensing. Back then, the elegant chestnut presented himself slightly unspectacular, but still let his quality shine through.

From then on, Herbert and Karin Rehbein assumed responsibility for Donnerhall's training. He turns out to be a model student, for whom everything just came together: willingness to perform, ride-ability, and first-class gaits predestined him for an international career in the dressage arena. In 1986, Donnerhall emerges as the winning stallion of the DLG-exhibition in Hanover (DLG = German Agricultural Society).

Donnerhall 2.5 years old, after his stallion licensing

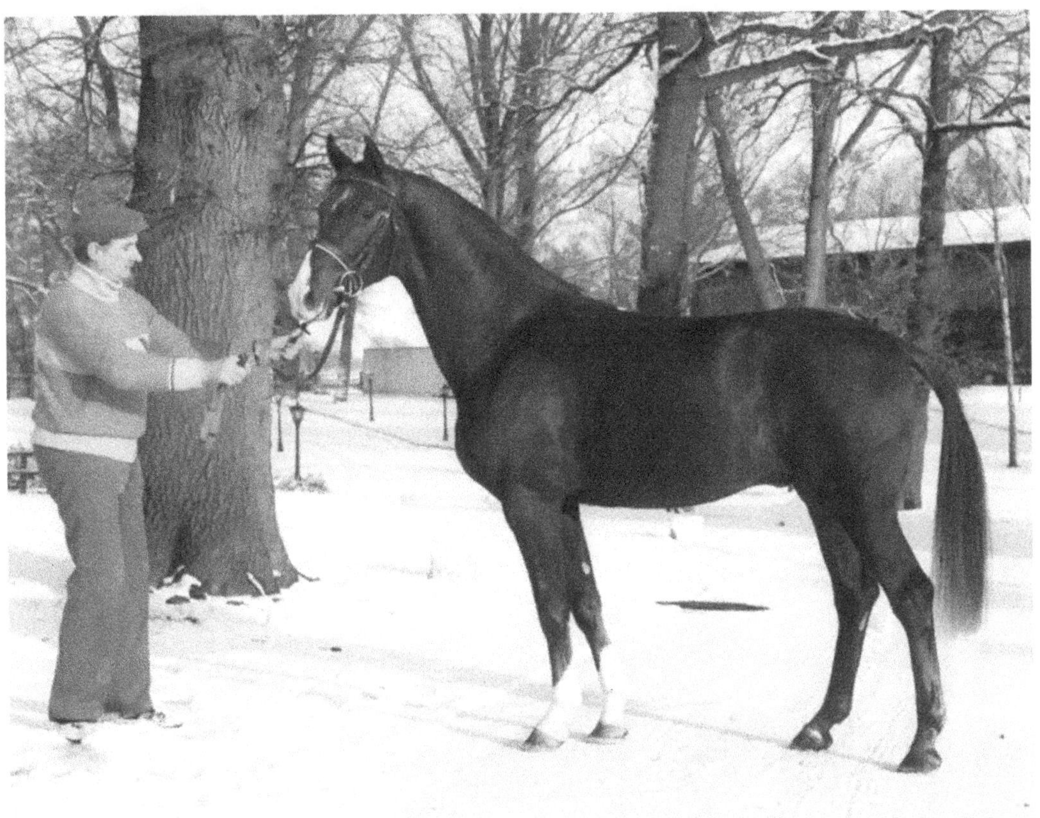

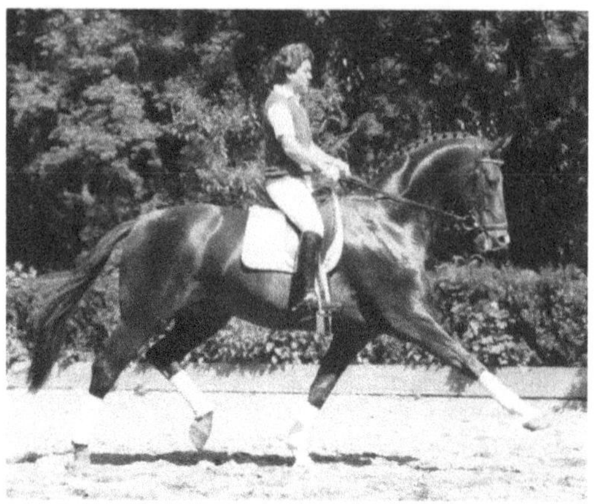

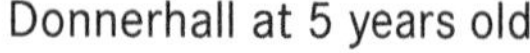

Donnerhall at 5 years old

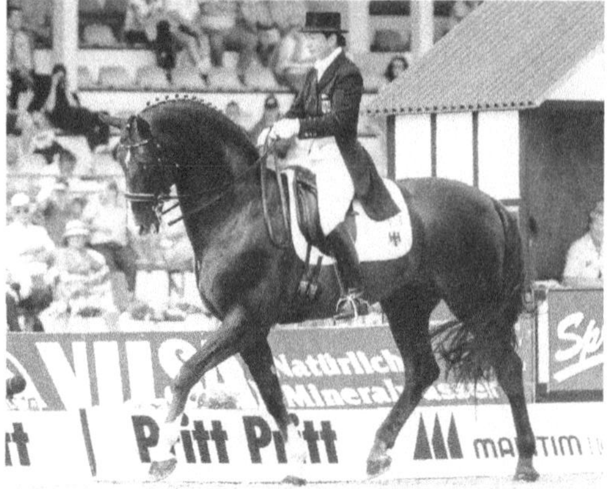

Donnerhall 16 years old–European Championships 1997 Verden

Success in dressage classes was not far behind. Donnerhall and Karin Rehbein manage to move up into the advanced levels of dressage, high placings and victories in Grand Prix and Grand Prix-Special classes follow.

They return with a team gold medal and individual bronze from the World Equestrian Games in Den Haag in 1994 and are also part of the winning team at the Europeans in Verden in 1997. In addition, they secure individual bronze. In 1998, the stallion is now 17, Karin Rehbein is once again part of the gold team at the World Equestrian Games in Rome and ranks an excellent 4th individually.

His skills as a sire are in no way inferior to his athletic performances: He can account for 121 licensed sons registered in the German Stallion Book No. 1, sired more than 1233 registered mares of which about 245 received the title of state premium mare. Numerous of his offspring are registered as sport horses. By now, Donnerhall is considered to be a line founder. The so called D-blood is firmly established in European horse breeding and is still much sought after.

In 2012, 10 years after his passing, offspring of this Oldenburg stallion of the millennium formed the entire German dressage team at the Olympic Games in the British capital:

Damon Hill – son of Donnerhall (Helen Langehanenberg)

Diva Royal – granddaughter of Donnerhall (Dorothee Schneider)

Desperados FRH – grandson of Donnerhall (Kristina Sprehe)

Frau Holle 17

Fürst Heinrich
Fürstenball
Maradonna
Bay | Mare | born 2012
Riccio
Rotkäppchen
Mona Lisa

In the year 2012, a very correctly built and remarkably beautiful filly by Fürstenball out of Rotkäppchen by Riccione was born at the facilities of Westphalian breeder Christoph Rawert. She distinguished herself by her sound character from a very early age: "Frau Holle has been very trusting and people-oriented from the beginning, but was still always alert and sassy", remembers her breeder from the German town of Coesfeld. She also proved her strong willingness to perform when she was first backed as well as during her basic training. Always easygoing and equipped with three good basic gaits, she received an overall score of 85% at the National Broodmare Show in Münster-Handorf in 2015. Test riders even awarded her 90% - further proof for the beautiful bay's motivation to work and willingness to learn.

Frau Holle led by her breeder Christoph Rawert at the German Elite Mare Championships in Lienen, 2015

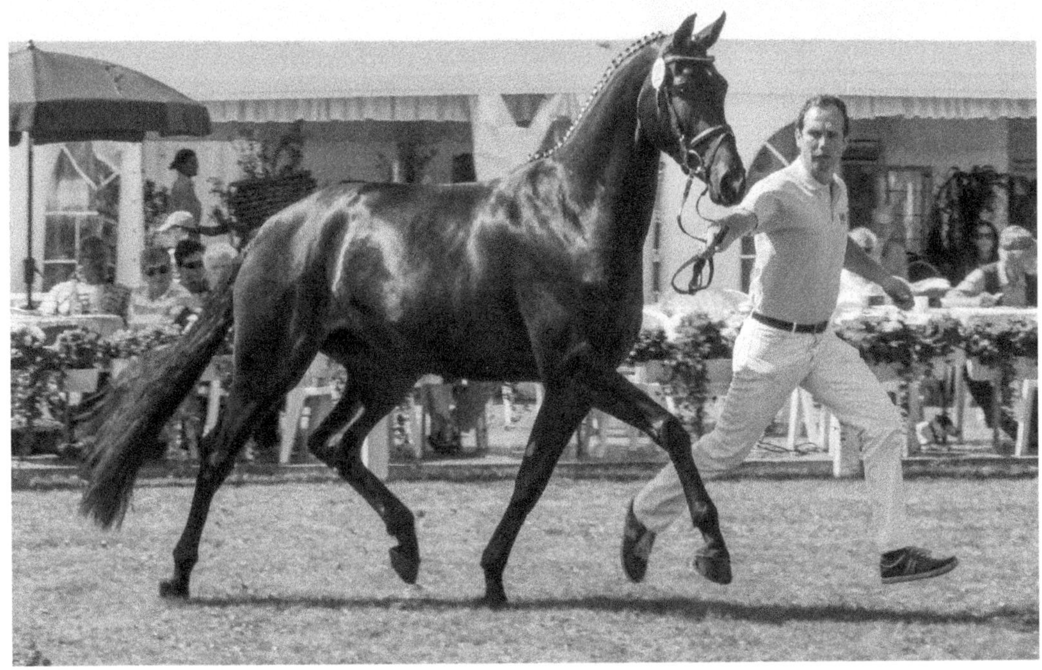

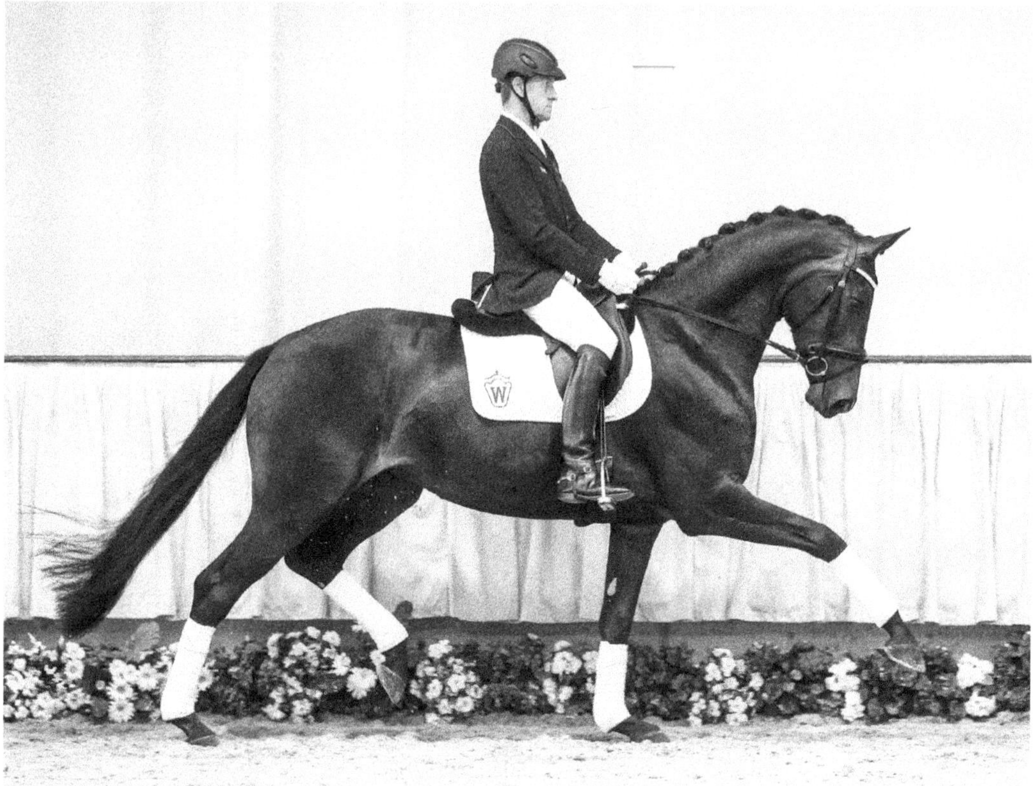

Frau Holle at 3 years old

As catalogue number 42, Frau Holle was sold as a 3-year-old at the Westphalian Elite Auction in Münster-Handorf in 2015. The auction catalogue describes the mare as follows: "Vater Fürstenball provides this likable state premium mare. An excellent dressage horse which demonstrates her perspective for the international sport by showing very good rhythm, suppleness, and a natural movement quality."

As a 6-year-old, she came under the saddle of Jana Schrödter: "She has already had placings in intermediate classes for young dressage horses. From the start, the mare showed to be very sensitive, eager, and willing to learn. However, she needed a bit of time to grow into her own big body. But with patience, calmness, and finesse, the lanky youngster developed more and more into a well-modulated and very motivated top athlete. Her extraordinary work attitude and the affinity to people of this special mare have helped us on our journey."

At 8 years old, the mare and rider Jana Schrödter, who had taken over the ride from her mother, won in a Prix St. Georg Special, a final qualifier for the Nuremberg Burg Pokal (Donaueschingen 2020). It can be clearly seen that the mare has continued to mature physically and is correctly muscled. Horse-appropriate and

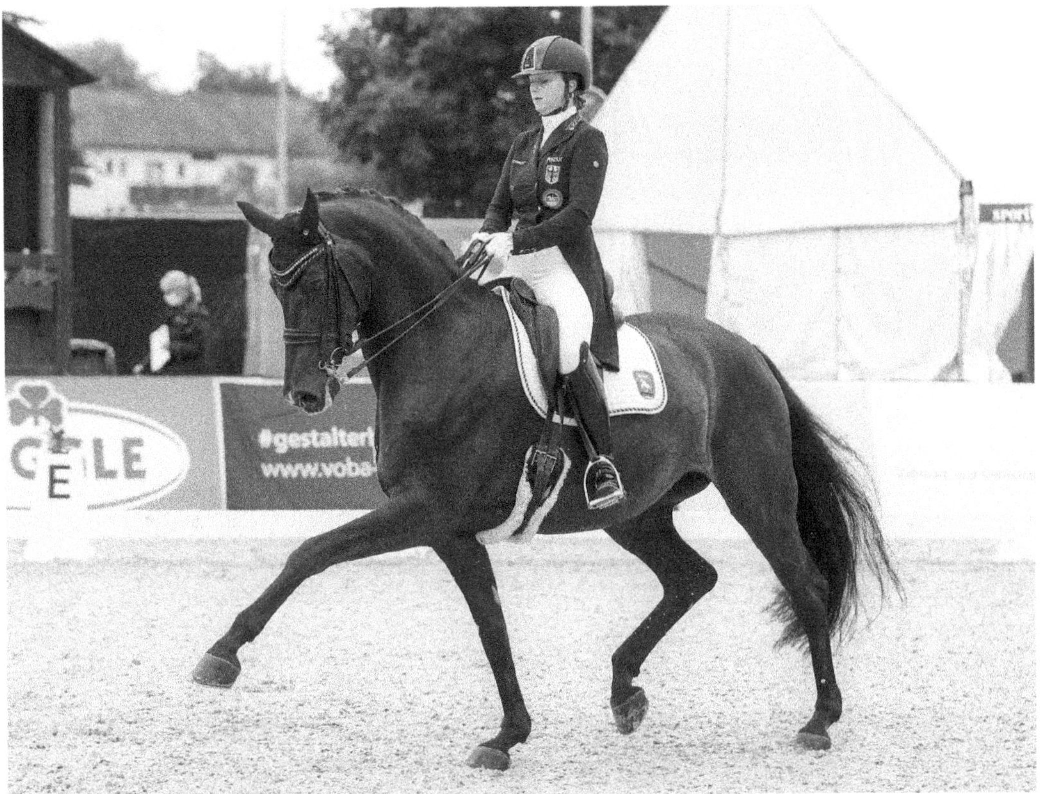

Frau Holle at 8 years old – Donaueschingen 2020

careful training has led the talented horse to high level athletic success, without having lost her eagerness, movement quality, and willingness to perform. The mare appears motivated and energetic, she stretches trustingly into her rider's hand with her ears pricked and a content expression on her face. "She has always strived to do everything right; in the beginning she was almost too motivated. It needed a few classes to fully bring her potential to the light."

1

General Notes on Muscle Function

The body's active organs of movement are the muscles which sensibly attach to two or more bones of the skeleton and extend across one or more joints. The musculoskeletal system is commonly described as being voluntary, i.e. subject to conscious control. This is only partially correct. It is true that a movement is initiated by a conscious decision, but the movement's pattern and a potentially subsequent complex chain of coordinated associated movements is carried out by a multitude of orderly reflexes but without the individual phases of this movement complex being consciously perceived. For the purpose of the following observations, we need only to concern ourselves with general postural reflexes, movement reflexes and postural movement reflexes. These form only a small part of the broad spectrum of independent reflexes. It suffices for the rider to know that the tonus* (the constant low-level activity of a body tissue, especially muscle tone) of individual muscles and of whole muscle groups is stimulated and maintained by reflexes. On the one hand, these reflexes are independent on body position (posture), but on the other hand, they are interdependent and largely interlinked. This results in an interdependence of the state of tension of several muscle groups, either directly or as an opposite effect (synergist – antagonist).

These interdependent relationships can be observed even more clearly on anatomical specimens of muscle tissue. The muscles of the limbs are divided into flexors and extensors according to their position in relation to the joints and their function. The function of the torso muscles cannot be so simply defined. These muscles are attached to large areas or in long rows to the torso bones and the function of several muscle groups is intertwined. Furthermore, many are joined by layers of connective tissue (fascia) and they are therefore dependent on each other to an even greater extent. This interdependence means that these large muscle groups must function in an organized interplay and that this is destroyed when just one of these large muscle groups is obstructed in its free, natural activity by the rider.

* the constant low-level activity of a body tissue, especially muscle tone - Editor's note.

Only the harmonious interplay of the entire body muscles will combine optimum performance with beauty of movement. The rider has to develop a feeling for this harmony and stimulate and maintain it during the training of the young horse, without obstructing or destroying it in any way. Only then will the rider be able to have their horse's movement and its four legs at their command by means of the aids the rider applies, as if horse and rider were one.

The very construction of the equine body predisposes the horse to be ridden. Its skeletal system has always been a suitable subject for research into the interrelation between form and function. The unilateral use of the movement apparatus to stand and to move forward in a more or less accelerated manner in a direction as straight as possible has led to significant adaptation of the skeletal frame to this type of function. In the case of the horse, its evolutionary history can be traced through analysis of archaeological findings in an almost unbroken line back to its ancestors which originally possessed an almost complete set of pedal bones with a subsequent gradual evolutionary reduction on the number of phalanges and metacarpal and metatarsal bones as well as the ulna and fibula.

In connection with the evolutionary reduction of certain bones of the limbs in equine ancestors to the very much simplified and strengthened form of today's horse, the active movement apparatus also had to change simultaneously in its form and function. These changes concern the position and internal structure of the muscles. It is unnecessary to go into detail as to the position; it will be fully described in the respective chapters. The changes which occur in the internal structure of the muscles affect the layout and corresponding number and length of the muscle fibers. There are muscles which are almost entirely composed of cells arranged parallel to each other (fleshy fibers); these fibers run through the entire length of the muscle in a more or less parallel direction (Figure 1). They taper swiftly toward the end, terminating in fine tendon fibers which, all together, form the much thinner tendon as compared to the muscle belly. This tendon is connected to the bone by being anchored firmly in the periosteum (membrane covering the bone). The function of such a muscle is to contract strongly and then relax, meaning they are passively stretched by opposing (antagonistic) muscles. These muscles are made up of long fibers and contract to a great extent because of the very considerable length of their constituent fibers (strong pulling action). They therefore produce movements with a strong thrust and

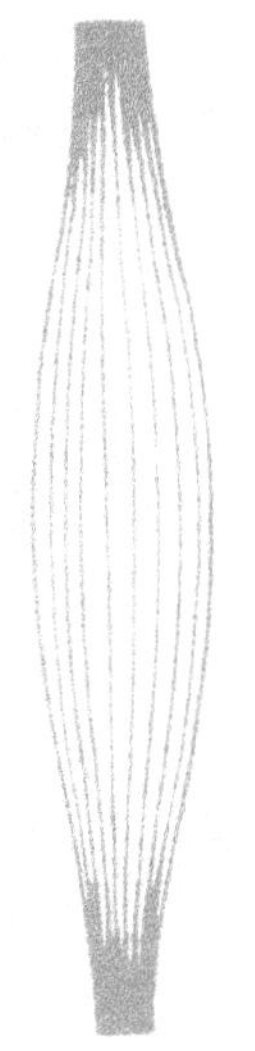

Figure 1: Muscle with long straight fibers

primarily serve to move forward. Fatigue substances (lactic acid) collect rapidly in these muscles when they are forced to remain contracted (tense). These muscles then swell as a result of lymphatic fluid in the surrounding tissue area and ache because of the subsequent pressure on the nerve endings. The more rhythmic the cycle of contracting and stretching, the better the circulation and, hence, the elimination of metabolic products, which also reduces the level of fatigue.

Other muscles are permeated by and covered to varying degrees by tendon fibers. The tendinous interspersion is present only at the beginning or end of the muscle; but they can also run through the entire muscle belly connecting the tendons at both ends across the muscle. These are tendinous cords which are sometimes quite thick or inlays in the form of squamous sheets. Indeed, an entire muscle might even change into a tendinous cord which acts solely and passively as a tension band and is of great importance for the position and support of the joints across which it extends whilst standing still or shifting weight during motion. In this function, the traction resistant tendon fiber takes over the purely passive function of carrying from the contractile muscle fiber. In the case of all these muscles which have special tendinous mechanisms, the contractile muscle fibers are not arranged parallel but obliquely to the lengthwise axis of the muscle. Therefore, the muscle fibers cannot permeate through the entire length of the muscle but skip from one tendinous segment to another. In this arrangement, each individual muscle fiber is shortened, however, the number of fibers in the muscle as a whole is increased by many times (Figure 2). As every muscle fiber of equal thickness produces equal force, irrespective of its length, it is understandable that in a muscle with such a quantity of tendinous inlay, the lifting force must be increased accordingly. The more work units (muscle fibers) are part of a muscle, (the larger the physiological cross-section), the stronger the muscle is.

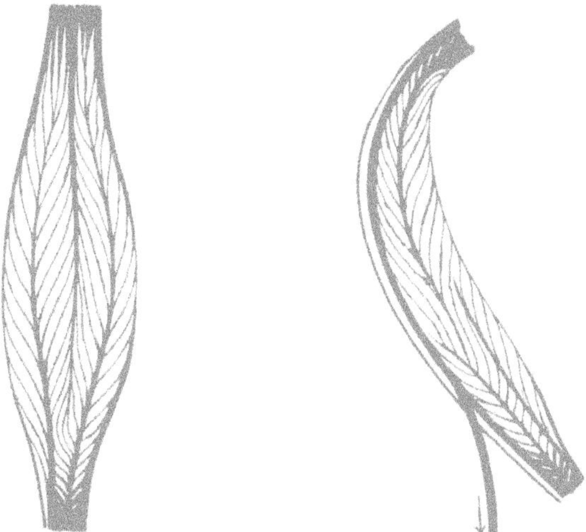

Figure 2: A muscle with oblique fibers and tendinous permeation (darker sections)
The 2nd picture shows the biceps muscle of the forearm (*M. biceps*), its oblique fibers with a continuous tendon, and the *Lacertus fibrosus* branching off from it.

It is assumed that these structural differences result in fundamental differences in performance. They are supposed to be the determining factor for speed and staying power (tempo and stamina) of racehorses in the sense that horses which have more tendinous fibers in their muscles have more staying power – they can gallop for longer periods of time – while others can be faster over a shorter distance but tire sooner. It must be pointed out, however, that there is no conclusive proof for this theory.

Knowledge of the anatomy of a muscle with reference to its position and inner structure makes it possible to ascertain its role. The shorter fiber muscles which are permeated with tendons can act as elastic supporting tensor bands for a long period of time. They do all of the work required for prolonged even tension or stretching. As static organs they enable the horse to hold itself in the position the rider asks for and take over the role of balancing the rider's weight. On the other hand, those muscles, which are composed mostly of long fibers without a permeation of tendons, are exclusively for forward movement, rapidly alternating between contraction and stretching. If these muscles are used for weight-bearing or holding a position for a long period of time, they will quickly tire, initially go into a state of cramped tension and then they will slacken and become flaccid.

There is a further function of the muscles of the limbs to which little attention has been paid thus far. During excessive strain, for example during the landing after a jump, the flexor muscles prevent an overextension of the joints, while the extensor muscles keep the open, elastic joints sufficiently flexed, prevent them from completely giving way, and, thus, allow the joints to take the entire strain and act as elastic springs. As opposed to actively contracting and stretching, this function is a passive or static use of the extensor muscles, bracing until they stretch. This is followed immediately by an active contraction of the muscle to continue the movement. This function is especially important for a riding horse when flexing the haunches and during landing after a jump.

Increasing muscular strength is synonymous with stimulating muscle growth. A muscle can grow through exercise only if it is used as nature intended according to its position and internal structure. However, it decreases in size (atrophies) if it is made to work in an incorrect, cramped tension which it cannot maintain long term. The resulting swelling and loss of muscle tone cause disturbances in the muscle's nutrition supply. Muscle mass is not replaced at the same rate as mass lost due to physiological degradation (wear and tear!), and the muscle consequently becomes smaller. **In contrast, muscles that work physiologically correctly, in a supple and rhythmic manner, have a good blood supply and are therefore better nourished. They are able to build new muscle fiber and become larger (increase their size as a result of work).**

These physiological findings are the basis for the following discussion of riding theory, intended to offer criteria beyond the principles of riding on how to train a horse, to identify and resolve riding problems as they arise, as well as encourage the development of muscle strength.

2

Why Do We Start Young Horses with the Neck Stretched Forward-downward?

a) Notes on Anatomical Function (see Figure 3 page 26 and Figure 4, page 33)

The horse's back is a bridge between the forehand and the hindquarters. We call it the **vertebral bridge** because it is composed of many individual bones, i.e. the vertebrae. The vertebrae are connected to each other by relatively immobile joints, strong ligaments, and discs of cartilage. These vertebrae are sub-divided according to their position in the horse's body as follows: the horse has 7 cervical vertebrae, 18 thoracic vertebrae, 6 lumbar vertebrae, 5 sacral vertebrae, and approximately 20 caudal vertebrae, of which the vertebrae of the sacral region have become fused together into one bone to form the sacrum. The sacrum is firmly attached to the pelvis by means of its lateral wings and numerous strong but elastic ligaments. It is here that the vertebral bridge receives the entire forward thrust from the hindquarters to transfer it along the back and transform it into forward movement.

Each pair of ribs is connected by a joint to each of the thoracic vertebrae. The horse therefore has 18 pairs of ribs. Of these, the first 8 are joined to the breastbone (sternum) by cartilaginous joints (true ribs). The remaining 10 are not joined to the breastbone (false ribs); their cartilaginous end sections meet and form the mobile arch of ribs. The true ribs, together with the breastbone, support the thorax. They have very limited mobility and enable the torso to be suspended on the forelimbs; they are therefore called **supporting ribs**. In contrast, the very mobile false ribs serve to extend the thorax and thereby facilitate breathing; they are called **breathing ribs**.

All the vertebrae of the back have ascending spinous processes of different length and angle. The spines of the front half of the back are angled toward the back, while those of the rear half point forward. The angle gradually decreases toward a middle vertebra whose spinous process is upright. The spines of the first vertebrae of the back, which number 12 on average, are of varying height and together form the foundation of the withers which progressively slopes down the back to disappear completely. The 5 spinous processes of the sacrum are angled backward unlike the processes of the rear half of the vertebral bridge which point forward. This indicates

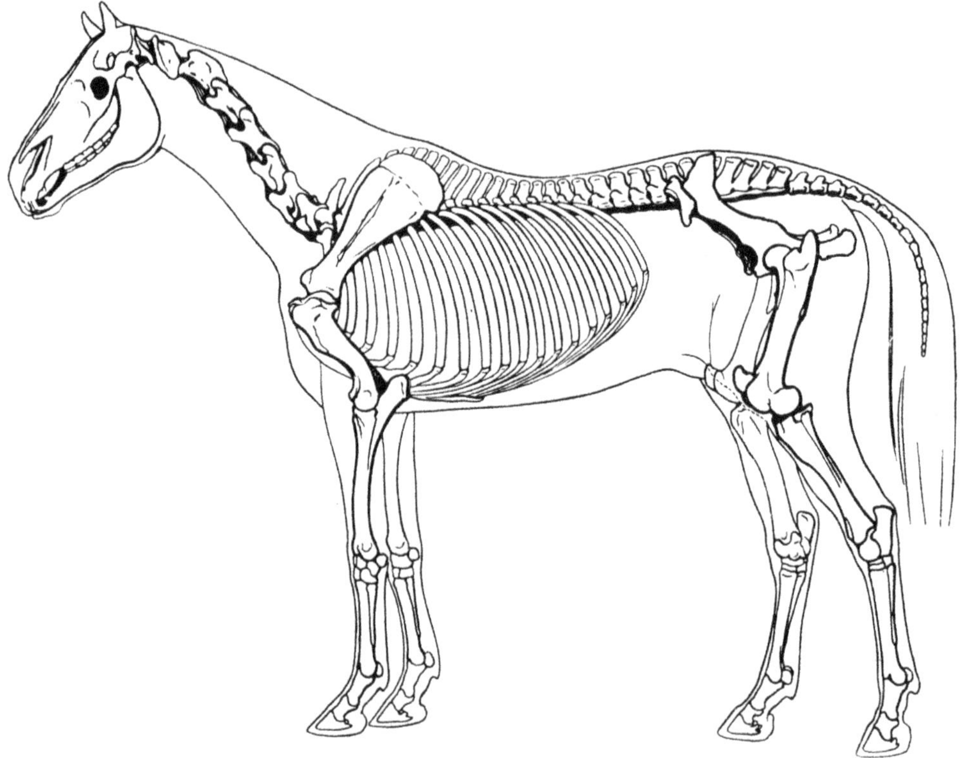

Figure 3: The skeleton of the horse

that the area has a different function: the sacrum acts as a counterfort[1], specifically as a support for the rear section of the vertebral bridge while another front counterfort can be perceived in head and neck.

The summits of all the spinous processes are connected by a tendinous ligament from which the nuchal ligament (**upper** brace of the vertebral bridge) extends up to the head. There is a further supporting mechanism in the form of the **lower** lengthwise brace, running from the front to the rear pillars of the bridge (forehand and hindquarters!). The mass of strong tendons of the abdominal wall, which are fused together into the white line in the middle, extend from the sternum backward to the front lower edge of the pelvic girdle (edge of the pubic bone). This mass of tendons can pull the sternum and pelvis against each other when contracted and thus offer further support for the bridge. **Zschokke**[2] (in personal communication) has proven that a fresh skeleton, from which all the muscles

[1] counterfeit: a buttress built against or integral with a wall (as a retaining wall or dam) but on the back or thrust-receiving side. Miriam Webster - Editor's note.

[2] *Anleitung zur Kenntniss und Gesundheitspflege des Pferdes,* Zürich 1910 (Instructions on horse knowledge and health care) Erwin Zschokke taught at the veterinary school in Zurich from 1877. After its incorporation into the University of Zurich as the Faculty of Veterinary Medicine in 1901, Erwin Zschokke was professor of veterinary medicine at the University of Zurich until his retirement in 1925. From 1905 to 1925 he was also director of the Zurich Animal Hospital. Erwin Zschokke was rector of the University of Zurich from 1916 to 1918. - Wikipedia - Editor's note

have been removed by dissection, leaving the ligaments intact, can still bear the weight of a heavy rider if the limbs have been secured in position. Relatively speaking, the back is least supported in the area of the lumbar vertebrae, and this is where its greatest mobility lies.

b) How Does the Horse Cope with the Rider's Weight?

When a young horse feels a rider's weight in its saddle for the first time, it usually arches its back and contracts it in a spasm; it turns into a humpback. Once it has calmed down, it rapidly relaxes and drops its back. If the horse is then led on, it walks unsteadily, also swaying from side to side under the weight, and the rider feels as if they were sitting in a rocking hollow. At this stage, the horse ultimately carries the weight solely with its skeleton, without the help of its muscles. It becomes obvious that the lower brace plays an important role in this because the horse, as it becomes progressively more tired, places its forelegs further forward and its hind legs further back (the horse is said to be strung out or disconnected). In the process, the ligaments of the lower bracing arch are passively tensed and placed under increasing strain without the contractile muscle fibers playing an active role. The horse is able to carry the rider for a certain time in this position, but its ability to move naturally is restricted. Once this position becomes uncomfortable for the horse, perhaps even causing back pain, it will initially try to stiffen and tense all of its back muscles (see Chapter 3) to be more able to carry the weight. The consequence of this stiffening is an unbalanced, tense movement with small steps and a hard, wooden feeling for the rider. It is difficult for the rider to "sit" into the movement of the horse. The long back muscle, which is relatively thick and fleshy with only superficial tendon cover on its outside, is not able to perform in a tense state for a long time; it will soon tire and become painful. As a result, the horse relaxes the back muscles, hollows it back, and drops it as in the beginning. This process can be continuously repeated. There may be horses which resign themselves to cope with the weight of the rider in this way for their entire lives. They will never attain a high level of performance or stamina. Their back does not swing, it is not supple. Such horses are uncomfortable; they do not let the rider sit and their trot is extremely bouncy.

Since we have ascertained that the long back muscle may not stiffen the vertebral bridge, we must conclude that it has a different role, and that carrying the rider's weight falls to other groups of muscles.

Some of the upper neck muscles, together with the nuchal ligament, have the task of maintaining the natural position of the back under the rider's weight (Figure 4, b, see Page 33). The summits of all of the spinous processes of the back are covered by a tendinous ligament which forms a broad cap on the withers. This ligament extends from the 3rd spinous process of the 3rd thoracic vertebra in the form of a strong elastic cord along the upper neck to the occipital bone. This nuchal ligament forms the base of the crest. An elastic *Lamina nuchae* composed of the same tissue extends from the nuchal ligament and the first spinous processes of the withers to the cervical vertebrae. On both sides of this sheet of nuchal ligament lie the muscles of the upper neck. They fill the large space between the cervical vertebrae and the nuchal ligament from the occipital bone to the withers and pull in the same direction as the nuchal ligament. There are several muscles which originate from different areas. To understand their function, it suffices to know that they are divided into two groups. The muscles of one group extend from the cervical and thoracic vertebrae to the occipital bone; they carry the head (Figure 4, a). The muscles of the other group extend from the dorsal vertebrae and the withers-shoulder sheet to the cervical vertebrae; they carry the neck (Figure 4, c and d). The deepest of these neck muscles, which supports the head (Figure 4, a) is permeated by tendon strips; therefore, it is, most of all, capable of operating continuously in a state of elastic tension. The strongest neck muscle is spleen-shaped (Figure 4, e) and extends from the withers and withers-shoulder sheet in a fan-like shape to the 5th to 3rd cervical vertebra and to the back of the head. It is entirely fleshy and carries out the large movements of the neck and head (Chapter 8).

Let us now look at the spinous processes of the withers. They are long and protrude from the front upward at an angle toward the back. They are therefore ideally positioned to act as the arm of a lever to produce a pulling action which is directed forward by the muscles of the upper neck. If the horse stretches its neck forward, the neck muscles and the nuchal ligament (Figure 4, b) exert a corresponding pulling action and the spinous processes of the withers become erect. This pulling action is directed onto the back by the tendinous ligament which, as direct extension of the nuchal ligament (Figure 4, b'), connects all spinous processes of the back and by the dorsal serrate muscle (Figure 4, f) which is split into many sections. This muscle is composed of many strips covered with tendinous layers which extend from each individual spinous process at an angle downward and backward along the arch of the dorsal and lumbar vertebrae, whereby they bypass two to six vertebrae. The strips are attached to the arches of the back and lumbar vertebrae in the same direction of pulling as the muscles of the upper neck are attached to the spinous processes. If the spinous processes are raised forward, the dorsal and lumbar vertebrae must follow forward and up. The back is thus raised, e.g., it returns to its natural position.

The trainer requires the rider to sit near the pommel of the saddle, as close to the highest point of the withers as possible. This is very important for the performance of the upper neck muscles, which support the rider's weight together with the arch of the back. This takes place through lever action. The distance between the withers and the rider (deepest point of the saddle) is the load-bearing arm, while the head and neck are the arm which transfers the force of the double-armed lever. The longer the force arm and the shorter the load-bearing arm, the easier it will be to bridge the load that is the rider's weight. Therefore, the rider must sit as far forward as possible and, in the case of young horses, further lighten the load on the horse's back by slightly leaning the upper body forward. With this extra help, the young horse will soon learn to balance the weight with the as yet untrained muscles of the upper neck and allow its neck to relax and drop. The horse should not let the possible excess weight or force exerted by a very long neck work to its disadvantage. If it does so, the horse becomes too low, leans on the bit, and it becomes extremely difficult to regain the required head-neck-carriage for riding. The horse should balance the weight of the rider with the weight of its head and neck – like a set of scales – whereby, in a "working" carriage, head and neck are simply suspended passively from the withers by the neck muscles and nuchal ligament. In such a position the muscles of the upper neck are stretched; the distance between the withers and the occipital bone – the force-transferring arm of the lever – becomes as long as possible. As a result, the neck takes on an upward convex shape and flexes in the throat latch, as the muscles in question are attached to the occipital bone. In this position, the back with the rider's weight on it attains its natural shape without any real active participation of the muscles of the upper neck. Only when an increased active elevation (relative raising of the forehand) is required of the horse in dressage, which results in a less efficient relationship between the force-transferring and load-bearing arms of the lever, do the upper neck muscles actively work to carry the back, i.e., they contract. Unfortunately, this elevation is accompanied by a shortening of the neck, which is why active elevation is frowned upon in everyday riding and also in dressage by many experts.

The muscles in the lower part of the neck which lower the head and the neck may not be assigned an active role. Mind you, the horse should let the head and stretched neck "drop," not actively bend and, in rider's parlance, not lean on the bit or come behind the bit and the vertical. It should stretch forward-downward seeking the rein from a giving hand and not remain in a bent position.

For the ridden horse, the head-neck-lever is the balancing pole which it uses to cope with the rider's weight in a way that leaves the muscle groups of the back and croup free to carry out their true function: **forward movement**.

c) Practical Application in the Training of the Young Horse

It is well known that horses with short or very well-muscled backs learn to stretch their necks much later or find it more difficult than horses with long backs or underdeveloped back muscle. The greatest degree of difficulty is posed by a well-muscled roached back if the neck is also short or thin. By contrast, horses with a poorly muscled, somewhat long or soft back (hollow back) very quickly learn to use their upper neck muscles. They tend to overdo this, to stretch the neck deep down and to lean heavily on the bit if the neck is sufficiently long and set broadly enough. If both these faulty types of back conformation are further compounded by a disproportionately short and light neck, these horses are not at all suitable as riding horses.

These practical observations can be easily explained. The short and well-muscled back is naturally able to carry considerable weight. The horse can carry the rider for long periods of time by alternating between tensing the vertebral bridge and sagging its back. The rider must very skillfully relax the muscles of the back and achieve contact despite a low neck (Chapter 3); whereas a horse with a weaker back tries to relieve its back much sooner and use the supporting muscles of its upper neck to carry the weight. Such horses often make faster progress in their training. Their backs improve visibly by the growth of the long back muscle as a result of training (Figure 4, g, see Page 33), while in the other type of horses a flattening of the back muscles can often be observed as a result of constant cramped tension. This cramped tension prevents sufficient circulation of blood in the muscle; the resulting excess fatigue substances inhibit the growth of new muscle mass. Since cells continually die and are renewed in the body, in this case growth, does not keep pace with degradation and the entire muscle diminishes in size.

The muscles of the upper neck can function as "static organs" for a long time without tiring significantly, but this needs a gradual increase in training. When young horses, after being ridden with a long and low neck for 20 to 30 minutes, suddenly lift the head and neck, tense or drop the back, it is not from ill will; these animals are suffering from neck pain brought on by fatigue. It is thus pointless to use force to correct this or to attach a side rein. One should rather address the cause, i.e., dismount and lead the horse for 5 minutes. Afterwards, the muscles are rested again, and in most cases, the problems have been resolved.

Nowhere is such substantial exercise-related growth of individual or groups of muscles more obvious as in the neck. One sometimes hears people say: "The muscles move from the bottom to the top." This is, of course, not the case. The muscles of the upper neck of a correctly moving horse are continuously made to work in their weight-bearing role and increase in size as any other working muscle does. The upper neck becomes broader; the triangle or hollow which can be seen in the young horse between the crest of the mane and the cervical spine fills out. By contrast, the muscles which flex the neck, hardly have an active role, do not become stronger, and even diminish in size. Consequently, the jugular groove on the lower part of the neck becomes ever more prominent.

The shape of the neck also changes over the course of training. The two supporting muscles of the neck lift the lower part of the neck with progressive growth due to training so that the concavity of this section balances out, the neck loses its S-shape, and a beautiful, evenly convex arch develops. The neck thereby becomes simultaneously longer.

An observant trainer can recognize whether their young horses are on the right track if the muscles are developing as described above.

3

The Back

(Figure 4, see Page 33)

In this chapter, we are going to focus on the long muscle of the back (Figure 4, g), one of the most powerful muscles of the body. It is composed of many layers of muscles arranged parallel to each other which are only covered with short end-tendon layers. These muscles exert a pull from the top rear toward the bottom front. The muscle originates at the back on the first spinal processes of the sacrum and the space between the sacral tuberosity and the coxal tuberosity[3] (hip bone) at the wing of ilium, as well as the spinous processes of the lumbar and last thoracic vertebrae and the strong aponeurosis (connective tissue) which covers the surface of the muscle in the lumbar region. The muscle bundles extend at an angle forward-downward and find their front point of action on all the thoracic vertebrae and the 7th cervical vertebra. If the muscle acts from rear base, it raises the forehand with an arched back. If the muscle contracts from its front point of action, it lets the back sag. When a horse tries to lighten the rider's weight on its back by contracting its long back muscle, it stiffens its back, does not swing, and does not let the rider sit.

The long muscles of the back on both sides do not function simultaneously during forward movement. When the supporting hind leg takes the weight of the horse's body, the long back muscle on the same side contracts from its rear point of action; at the same time the diagonal foreleg swings forward. In this manner, the long muscle of the back, together with the large gluteal muscle, relieves the forehand during motion. This function is at its highest perfection in canter because the muscles of both sides, enveloped in fascia which meet in the middle over the spine, work together in the same spirit, and because the alternating rhythm of contracting and stretching of muscles is more efficient in canter. All riders know that the fastest method of suppling horses with a stiff back is to ride frequent trot to canter transitions and that extensive canter work is the best way to strengthen a poorly muscled back. In trot, the long back muscles operate in the opposite way. One can recognize this by the

[3] The coxal tuberosity is the lateroventral projection of the wing of ilium. It is an important landmark : it forms the points of the hip visible in the horse and ox and palpable in the dog. - vet-Anatomy. - Editor's note.

alternate swelling and flattening of both sides. If the right muscle behind the saddle is at its highest arch, the left is flat, i.e., stretched. The greatest degree of extension occurs when the hind leg on the same side is swinging forward. The most arched point of the muscle – equalling the most contracted – on the other side, can be seen, when the hind leg on the same side has been set on the ground and is supporting. Hence, the side of the supporting hind leg is arched and the side of the swinging leg is stretched. The alternate lifting of the forehand therefore immediately follows after the hind leg on the same side is set on the ground and practically coincides with the moment the diagonal foreleg swings forward (see Chapter 4).

Only a well-trained back is also able to raise the forehand in trot. This is why the swinging back and the horse allowing the rider to sit to the medium and extended trot is the touchstone of a well-ridden horse. The so-called "high speed" at which the rider is lifted out of the saddle in medium trot is not an inalterable quality of a horse, but, in fact, the direct consequence of a rigidly tense back which does not swing. By raising the forehand the horse's movements become elevated and cover more ground.

A section of the large gluteal or croup muscles (Figure 4, l) originates in the fascia – a rough tendinous cover on the surface of the long back muscle. Thus, both of these muscles are coupled together during movement, which means that the hind legs cannot step freely forward in a relaxed manner if the back is rigidly tense and cramped. Conversely, the back muscle cannot function unhindered if the hind legs are hindered in their natural rhythmic movement by the rider (incorrect leg and rein aids!). The fascia of the back and lumbar region covers both muscles. The broad back muscle extends from the fascia (Figure 4, h) and runs from the lumbar and rear back area in the form of a broad sheet at an angle across the ribs to the upper arm. If the long back muscle is in cramped tension, this state is also transferred to the broad back muscle. This restricts the upper arm and hinders the forward stride of the foreleg. The horse then has a restricted gait. Freedom in the shoulder can only be achieved through suppleness of the back and the broad back muscle. The long back muscle is also attached to the ribs. As long as it is tense, it inhibits the horse's breathing. As soon as it gives up its cramped tension and swings rhythmically, the horse can breathe freely and snorts. From experience, snorting indicates that a horse is becoming supple. It is the incorrect seat of the rider which first and foremost hinders the function of the back muscles. The seat of a rider pounding down on the long back muscle in trot forces this muscle into spasmodic tension. The rider should sit lightly into the horse in a forward motion, i.e., in the direction of the fibers of the long back muscle. The back will supple even quicker if less weight is placed on it and the rider sits carefully in the saddle. Therefore, the rider should always commence a training session in rising trot and only go into sitting trot when the horse lets them sit, i.e., when the back is swinging with suppleness.

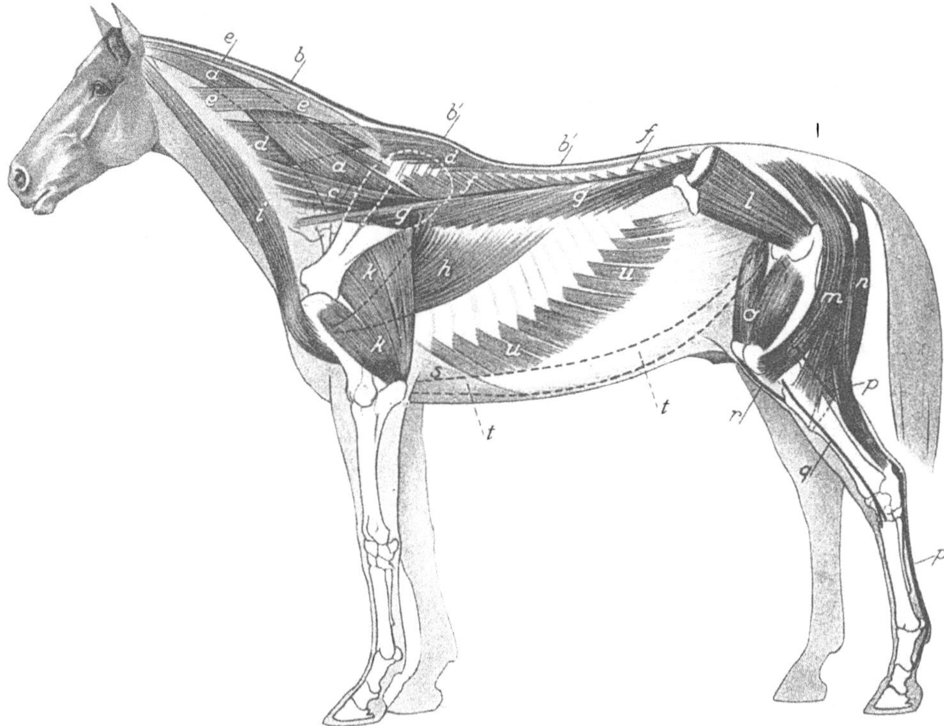

Figure 4: The important muscles of the neck, back, and the hindquarters of the left side of a horse from the rider's point of view. Some of the superficial muscles are deliberately shown smaller than their true size so that the deeper muscles become visible.

a Supporting muscle of the head, *M. semispinalis capitis*

b, b' Nuchal ligament

c+d The long supporting muscles of the neck, namely

c long neck muscle, *M. longissimus cervicis*

d withers' muscle, *M. spinalis*

e Spleen-shaped muscle, *M. splenius*

f Dorsal serrate muscle, *M. multifidus*

g Long back muscle, *M. longissimus dorsi*

h Broad back muscle, *M. latissimus dorsi*

i Head-neck-arm muscle, *M. brachiocephalicus*

k Extensor of the elbow, *Mm. anconaei*

l Large gluteal muscle, *M. glutaeus medius*

m Lateral long muscle of the ischium, *M. biceps femoris*

n Caudal long muscle of the ischium, *M. semitendinosus*

o Supporting muscles of the patella and extensors of the stifle joint, *M. quadriceps femoris*

p+q The tendinous connection between stifle and hock joints, namely

p the almost entirely tendinous superficial digital flexor (flexor of the 2nd phalanx), *M. flexor digitalis pedis superficialis*

q flexor of the hock, part of the stay apparatus/flexor tendon of the foot, *Tendo femoro tarseus*

r Stifle joint/patella

s Deep thorax-humerus muscle, *M. pectoralis humeri ascendens*

t Straight abdominal muscle, *M. rectus abdominis*

u External oblique abdominal muscle, *M. obliquus abdominis externus*

In conclusion: The long muscle of the back (Figure 4, g) is clearly a muscle of movement, whose function is **exclusively forward movement and not to carry the weight of a rider**. It is connected by the broad back muscle (Figure 4, h) and large gluteal muscle (Figure 4, l) to the fore and hind limbs, and it is thus engaged in the rhythm of movement. Free, ground-covering, and rhythmic gaits are only possible if the long back muscle swings naturally and elastically without being restricted by the rider and their weight. Thus, the primary goal at the beginning of a training session is to achieve a supple back. Over the course of a horse's entire training, a systematic training of the back muscles is required (transitions to canter, long canter sessions while hacking out, climbing hills). The canter is much more important and builds much more strength than the trot. The trainer must pay special attention to the development of the flat back muscles in the young horse, which should become rounded over the course of its training. The play of the supple back muscles should be clearly visible in the rhythm of the movement.

4

The Hindquarters

a) Notes on Anatomical Function (Figure 4, see Page 33)

Nature has created the forehand to carry weight and the hindquarters for forward thrust. Accordingly, there is a significant difference in how the forehand and the hindquarters are connected to the torso. There is no osseous connection between the forehand and the thoracic cage (rib cage). Rather, the thoracic cage is elastically suspended between the shoulders of the forelimbs by a strong muscle, the suspensory muscle of the torso, which extends from the inner surface of the shoulder blades from above in a fan-like shape down to the supporting ribs and the end of the neck. This acts as a natural suspension for the forehand, whatever the position of the limbs. The hind leg is connected at the hip with the pelvis and therefore with the torso through joints. Thus, the elastic hindquarters required of the riding horse can only be achieved by flexing all the joints of the limbs in motion. This "flexed gait" is extremely demanding on the muscles because it means that the supporting limbs must be held in a slightly bent, elastic position in the very moment when the greatest strain is placed on them (in the supporting phase). The rider calls this active elastic function of the hind legs, the flexed gait, "flexing of the haunches." As this is extremely strenuous for the horse, 90% of all difficulties when riding are to be found here. The existence of very strong muscles with hardly any tendinous tissue interspersed, as well as entirely tendinous ligament structures with purely static function make it easier for the horse to use its hindquarters in this way. On the other hand, the suspension in the joints during movement requires less muscular activity with the help of the same (static) apparatus, the greater the angle of flexion remains, i.e., the closer the joints are in the extended position. The strain placed on the muscles increases in proportion to the degree of flexion of the joints. The accuracy of this observation can be confirmed by carrying out squats of varying height yourself. Therefore, all horses tend to hold their hip, stifle (anatomically speaking: the knee), and hock joints as extended as possible.

The muscles of the hindquarters of the horse have to fulfill **two roles**:

1. to push off from the ground in the natural forward movement,
2. to carry elastically with flexed haunches (suspension).

It is essential to set out these fundamental concepts of riding to understand the following explanation of anatomical function.

All the joints of the hind legs are not supported vertically but angled in such a way that they should buckle when standing. Without anatomical knowledge, one can consider this angled position to be unsuitable for an animal which is supposed to carry loads. This is, however, not the case for a horse which is moving freely. The stifle and hock joints are connected to each other by two entirely tendinous ligament structures (Figure 4, p and q) in extension and flexion in such a manner that extending or flexing the stifle automatically initiates the same movements in the hock joint and vice versa. Furthermore, when it is in full extension, the patella (kneecap, referred to as the stifle in English) is supported on a protruding nose of the femur and thus locks the joint in position. The patella is held in place by the extremely strong and fleshy femur (thigh) muscle (Figure 4, o). The hock is simultaneously fixed in an extended position by the brace of its tendon. Hardly any muscular strength is required to maintain this delicate balance. Conversely, the hip joint does not possess a similar brace. Hence, these are the only muscles which tire in a standing horse without any weight on its back.

The enormous muscle mass of the hindquarters is divided into four groups according to its position on the parts of the skeleton:

1. the croup muscles (gluteal muscles)
2. the inner loin muscles
3. the long muscles of the ischium
4. the supporting muscles of the patella or extensors of the stifle

Their function is dependent on the movement sequence and can vary in one and the same muscle.

The **croup muscles** originate on the pelvis and sacrum. They are attached to the femur in the area of the hip joint. The femur bone possesses lever-like bone processes to which the muscles are attached. Two of these processes are positioned below the hip joint, another forms the extension of the femur across the joint in an upward direction. The gluteal muscles, which are attached to the process above the joint, are therefore extensors, while the others are flexors of the hip joint. Extensors are considerably stronger than flexors. The latter act on the swinging leg and therefore do not have to overcome much resistance. The hip joint extensors have two tasks: firstly, to push the supporting limbs off the ground to move forward and secondly, as a static function, to maintain the flexed position of the hip joint of the supporting leg as the haunches are bent as is required in dressage.

The largest of the gluteal muscles (Figure 4, l), the main extensor of the hip joint, originates in part on the fascia of the long back muscles in the loin region. Consequently, both these muscles work in tandem and forcibly in the same rhythm. While the haunches are flexed, the gluteal muscle which is extended by the flexing of the hip joint pulls on the long muscle of the back and works together with this muscle to take the weight off the forehand. If the long back muscle is not uninhibited to carry out this function, but has it become rather tense by having to bear weight incorrectly, it cannot follow the pull of the large gluteal muscle. Thus, the forehand is not raised, the gaits can never become elevated and extended, and the movement of the horse can never become rhythmic.

The **inner loin muscles** extend from the lower surface of the spine to the pelvis and to the inner side of the femur. Together with the superficial gluteal muscles, they swing the hind leg forward and are therefore the flexors of the hip joint. In canter, they are also able to pull the whole pelvis forward, together with the abdominal muscles. As a result of this pulling action, in horses with a good canter, the back takes on the form of an upward bent bow during the moment of suspension when the hind legs are brought far forward. Conversely, the loin muscles make the back sag downward in incorrect and undesirable tension.

The three **long muscles of the ischium** (Figure 4, m and n) completely fill the rear section of the femur. They originate on the sacrum and the ischial tuberosity, generally speaking in the rear section of the croup. They loop around the back of the hip joint toward the stifle, which they effectively encompass from behind and above when the horse steps forward and under its body. Their entire pulling action begins at the stifle and acts in a backward direction. The stifle joint of the supporting leg is pulled backward by the contraction of the long muscles of the ischium which extends the angle of the stifle joint. Because of the tandem action described above, this extension of the stifle is synonymous with the extension of the entire limb in the same way it occurs in the pushing-off phase of each step. Consequently, the function of these muscles is exactly the same in respect to forward movement as that of the large gluteal muscle. The pull of the accessory tendon to the point of the hock functions in the same manner as it simultaneously produces the extension of the hock.

The **supporting muscles or extensors of the stifle joint** (Figure 4, o), are positioned on the front of the femur between the ilium and the patella. Their names indicate their role. As the leg pushes off the ground, they act as extensors of the stifle joint; as the haunches flex, they offer support to the patella. They therefore contribute in considerable measure to the flexed gait.

During flatwork, a horse is not only required to push off strongly but to flex its haunches, i.e., the flexed gait in the supporting phase. It is the combined function of all the **extensor muscles** to maintain this. In the process, several muscles combine efforts with the tendinous ligament structures which link the stifle and hock joints (Figure 4, p and q). Herein lies their static function. One has to emphasize again that the patella is steadied in an extended position on the *Trochlea* of the femur; the stifle and hock joints are thus locked without great muscular effort: the limb is rigid except for the hip joint. When the horse puts weight on the limbs as it flexes the haunches, the patella, as the upper point of the brace, is mobile. The patella with its straight ligaments (Figure 4, r) and the tendinous ligament structures of the stifle and hock joints (Figure 4, p and q) are only gaining hold on the supporting apparatus of the patella and in their connection with the long muscles of the ischium. This hold, however, is elastic, automatically producing an elastic effect in both joints as far as the extensor muscles allow, which are now acting as muscular tendinous ligament structures. It is this static use of all the extensor muscles which needs much more effort and requires lengthy training as opposed to pushing off from the ground with rapidly alternating contraction and extension.

All the muscles that have been referred to here which are used for forward thrust and the elastic flexed gait are predominantly fleshy; they have very little or no tendinous reinforcement. It then becomes understandable why nearly all horses stubbornly resist flexing their haunches as this demands a great deal of muscular effort.

b) The Sequence of Movement of the Hindquarters

The movement of the hind leg has four phases which are swinging forward, setting down on the ground, supporting, and swinging off the ground, or rather pushing off. These sequences are the same in every gait. When one watches a young horse moving freely, one can observe the following: the hind leg swings forward in a flexed position; at the moment of setting down on the ground, the hip joint is flexed to the maximum, however, the stifle and hock joints are not fully extended. At the moment when the supporting leg takes the weight of the body, the entire limb flexes slightly but elastically in all its joints. Only then does the limb begin to extend in all its joints and it attains the maximum degree of extension as it pushes off. **It is the fundamental prerequisite of training to preserve this natural movement in the young horse.** Everything else such as carriage and rein contact is of secondary importance; if these are given precedence during training, it will cause problems sooner or later if the natural sequence of movement is destroyed as a result. This natural movement is rhythmic and, therefore, the rider should first and foremost pay attention to the rhythm of the movement.

But, what happens in the hind leg if the movement loses its natural quality? The most strenuous part is the one-time elastic flexion action, i.e., the flexion of all joints in the supporting leg. The aim of the rider is to consciously feel this phase, to prolong it, and, thus, to give more impulsion to the movement. Understandably, the horse would rather shorten or exclude this phase completely because taking on weight in the extended position requires less muscular effort. The horse is able to keep its joints in the extended position during the supporting phase if it limits the action of its hind legs, i.e., takes shorter steps. If the steps are shortened in the back, hence the limbs come off the ground too early, then the horse displays a restricted movement, or it "hurries" with short steps, ("runs away under the rider"). If the steps at the front become shorter as the limbs are set down too early, the rider has the feeling that the horse becomes taller behind the saddle; the horse is only pushing off and falls on the forehand. The horse's step can only cover ground with the phase of flexing the haunches, as the other hind leg then has time to swing forward.

But what is the reason that the horse loses its natural movement? This is always the fault of the rider! Those who are honest have to admit that these movement difficulties first occur in the training of young horses when they take up rein contact, and the difficulties increase to a frightening extent with mediocre riders when double bridles are used.

The rein aid is a regulating aid which, if used correctly, does not limit the range of forward movement of the hind leg but its forward thrust and momentum (see Chapter 7 b). The full-halt, or rather half-halts for preparation, must be applied in the rhythm of the movement of the hind limbs, exactly in the moment of flexing the supporting leg. This means that the half-halts must act alternately on each leg and are immediately released once this leg begins to push off from the ground. Thus, the phase in which the joints are flexed is prolonged at the expense of the pushing off phase, the forward thrust (pushing off) is limited, and the horse steps – so to speak – into the (half-)halt. The rider has the feeling that the horse becomes bigger in front during the halt. In young horses, the full halt must be used very carefully; the rider must initiate it with great sensitivity and release it gradually in the rhythm of the movement to avoid damaging untrained muscles. A good rider maintains constant rein contact while riding a halt which is perfectly co-ordinated with the rhythm of the horse's movement. This halt is the natural consequence of a correct seat. The mistake which is most frequently made is that the rider simply continues to pull on the reins, i.e., senselessly pulls without using driving aids at the same time. Horses will react differently according to their disposition, but all horses will avoid flexing the hind leg. Some push off more strongly and lean on the bit, thus becoming faster; others move their heads about so that rein contact is lost and finally somehow come to a halt, usually halting abruptly with their forelegs so that the rider falls forward.

What has been said about the full halt, also applies to the use of the reins during movement. An insensitive backward-acting hand puts too much strain on the supporting flexed hind leg and teaches the horse to evade this position. As a result, its steps will inevitably become shorter, as described above. As the horse learns to resist the rein aids, it loses trust and naturalness; it will be wary of inept rein aids and will not find its natural rhythm.

The movements of the high school, piaffe and passage, are the very embodiment of perfect flexion in the haunches. The phase in which the supporting leg is flexed is as long as possible; in fact, it almost becomes a rocking movement. As the leg is extended to push off the ground, this is no longer a gradual movement of dragging the joints; it suddenly becomes an energetic movement out of the flexed position: pushing off from the ground acquires a quality of impulsion. The other hind leg can be encouraged to step far forward during the prolonged supporting phase. The movement with impulsion is therefore also ground-covering. When the haunches are flexed, the horse appears to grow in front; in reality, the croup is lowered. The extended trot is one of the most difficult movements in dressage tests. It is only correctly ridden if there is an obvious flexion in the haunches during the supporting leg phase and the horse swings the leg off the ground so energetically that there is a moment of suspension above the ground as in canter (Figure 5) and the rider sits deeply in the saddle as if glued to it. A high level of training and throughness is required if pushing off from the ground is not to win the upper hand compared to flexion of the haunches, in which case the elevated quality of the movement would be lost.

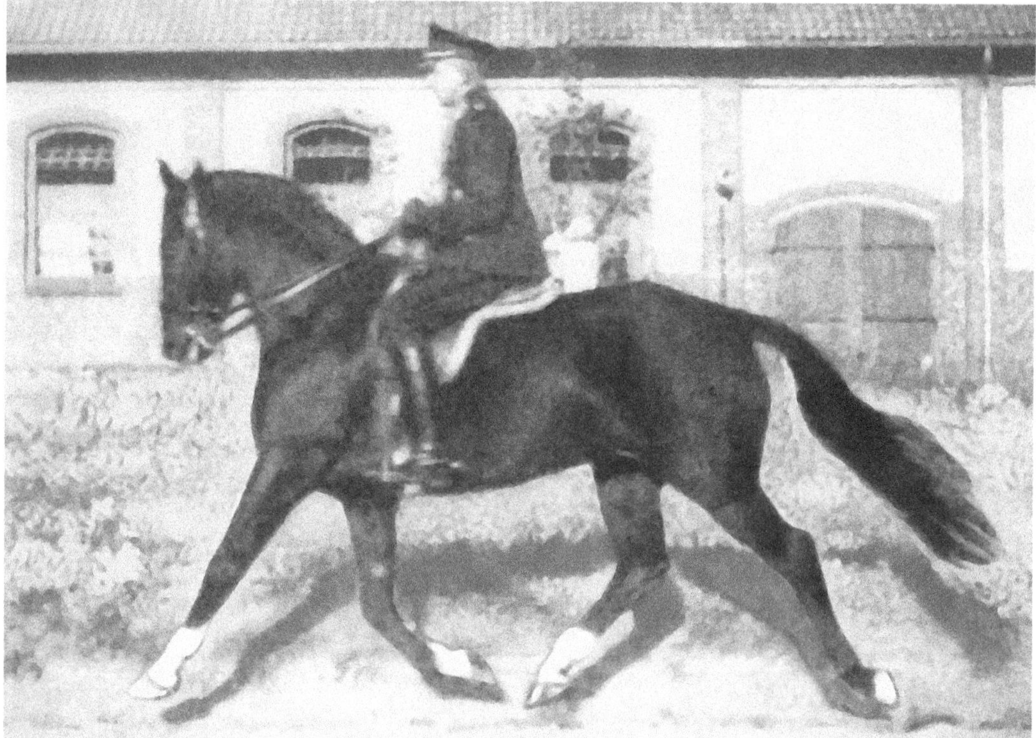

Figure 5: Moment of suspension in extended trot

The situation in the canter is no different. A pronounced phase of flexing the haunches is followed by an energetic swinging off from the ground and results in a ground-covering, elevated canter stride. If the hind legs are rather extended, the canter stride is short and flat above the ground. Such horses "roll over the forehand" and usually become heavy in the hand. The (half-)halt must be applied immediately after the inside hind foot has been set down on the ground, i.e., in the flexion stage of the haunches, if it is to be effective. If it meets the extending legs in the moment in which they are pushing off, the effect will be even more counter-productive than in the trot. Highly spirited horses will most likely lean on the bit, take away the rider's rein aids, and they will often bolt.

We should be aware here of a misleadingly incorrect phrase in common use. It is always said that "a horse should step far under its centre of gravity." This in itself is not sufficient. Of course, it should step as far forward as possible with the swinging leg, but the supporting leg must simultaneously be in the flexion phase. Only then do the hindquarters carry so much of the entire body weight that the forehand can swing forward in elevated steps at the correct moment. If the supporting leg evades the flexion phase, the croup will almost be lifted over the extended leg, the whole weight falls on the forehand, and the supporting leg remains planted on the ground for a longer period of time. The result is that the hind leg which has stepped far under the horse's body has to step next to the front foot or the horse overreaches. It can be easily proven that stepping far under is in itself useless if one "collects" a horse which is not through in the halt by using excessively strong rein and leg aids. The horse reacts by placing both extended hind legs far under its body. In this position, it is firmly planted on the ground like a sawhorse and can, for example, resist rider's aids to make it step backward just as if its legs were extended in a backward direction; at the least, it will sooner "rear" than step backward.

c) Application in the Training of the Young Horse

The most important rule is to retain the horse's natural movement. As speed and length of steps and strides vary from horse to horse, at first one should not ride together with other horses in a single file ride with certain spaces between horses. The horses first have to learn to go forward willingly in response to the leg aids; the use of the whip immediately after applying the leg is helpful. The rider has to develop a feeling for the horse's individual, natural movement and notice whether the horse is holding back or hurrying and accordingly either use stronger leg aids or use the rein to bring the horse back without a classic half-halt. In this preliminary stage, riding is rather a lesson in obedience than training. The horse will be encouraged by the driving aids to develop its natural free movement into an active forward movement. If the horse is moving actively and **purposefully forward**, it stretches of its own accord and seeks rein contact. The rider should accept this contact. This is the very moment when the rider can begin to influence the hind leg with regulating aids, making it flex its haunches. This must be done very carefully but consistently (see Chapter 7); the purity and the rhythm of the movement must be retained, and the horse must be willing to go forward instantly in response to more strongly applied driving aids and a giving hand and it should never retract independently. Changes of speed within each of the gaits and "fading" halts have the best gymnastic effect on the hindquarters. Frequent and lengthy periods of canter, if possible while hacking out, are essential to develop forward thrust. As we know, the same muscle groups are responsible for flexion in the haunches and forward thrust. This explains why it has been proven that alternating between riding in the school and hacking out and climbing hills (Figures 6 and 7) is the most effective way to develop the hindquarters. They complement each other; one is a gymnastic training of the horse's dexterity, the other builds up the horse's strength. Both are necessary.

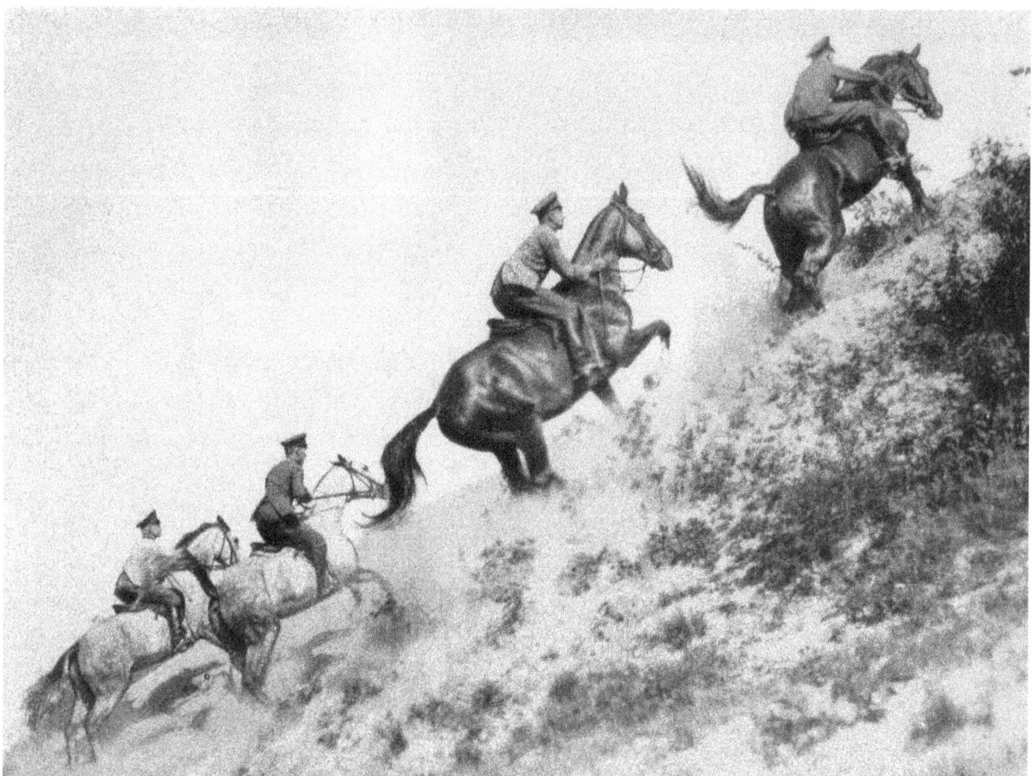

Figure 6: Climbing uphill. The rider at the front is climbing correctly in walk. This is an excellent method of training which uses and strengthens all the muscles. Climbing uphill in canter is much easier for the horses, and therefore, not as effective as a training method.

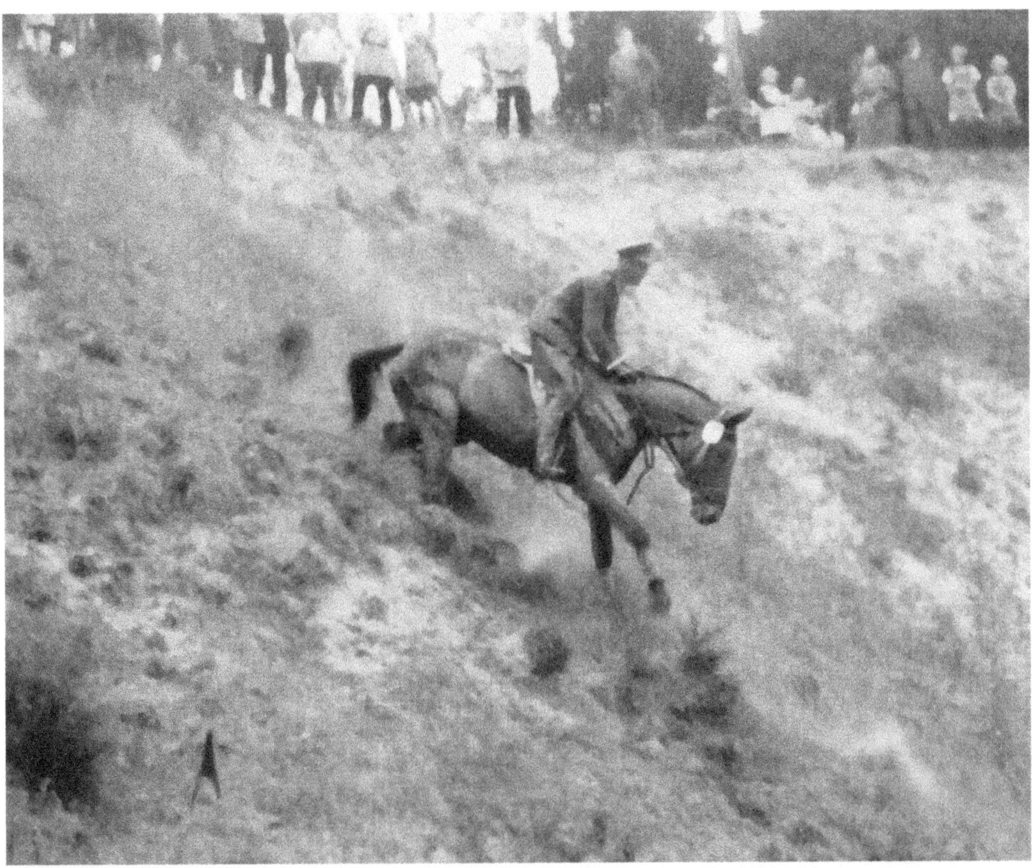

Figure 7: Riding downhill in walk, a particularly good method of training muscles of the hindquarters for flexing the haunches.

5

The Forehand

a) Notes on the Anatomical Function (Figure 8, see Page 47)

The forehand must be discussed from quite different perspectives than the hindquarters and the other parts of the body. The hind leg, back, abdominal muscles etc. develop through movements and levels of strength which are proportionate to their performance capability. Damage to their active organs of movement (muscles, tendons) very rarely results from overexertion because horses tire first, and accordingly try to conserve energy before an injury occurs. (We are not referring here to conditions of the skeleton as a result of conformation faults).

An active development of power (pushing off, swinging off) is also present in the forehand, however, in the riding horse, this is of secondary importance to the passive stress on the forehand when absorbing impact, acting as springs, balancing, and supporting the body during movement and especially during landing after a jump. This is what nature intended that the forehand do. This is why, from experience, a strong forehand is imperative for a future riding horse. Everything else can be strengthened and formed through correct training without any danger of injury to the horse. This also applies to the forehand, but it is more likely that the forehand, which is relatively weaker than the rest of the body, will suffer injury to the tendons or joints. Statistically, there is a greater incidence of medical conditions affecting the forehand than the hind legs. Hence, stability is the deciding factor. To what extent this is dependent on the skeleton as well as position and angle of the limbs can be found in textbooks on the horse's conformation. This book is only concerned with the muscles and tendons and their use in a functional context.

It is a well-known fact that the horse's forelegs do not tire when it is standing, whereas the hind legs do, and are, therefore, alternately rested. It is necessary to explain this aspect in detail because it is important not only with reference to standing.

The flexor tendons are stretched taut while the horse is standing. The deep digital flexor tendon (Figure 8, a') is connected by tendinous ligament structures (carpal check ligament, Figure 8, a") to the palmar surface of the carpal joint (knee). The superficial digital flexor tendon (Figure 8, b') receives an identical radial check ligament (Figure 8, b") above the joint. Thus, the flexor tendons in conjunction with the check ligaments form a completely autonomous tendon apparatus which carries or holds the foot and digital joints under the weight of the body without any muscular activity. The suspensory ligament with its tendinous structure (Figure 8, c, c'), made up of the *M. interosseus medius* (Figure 8, c) and the distal sesamoid ligaments of the proximal sesamoid bones (Figure 8, c'), supports the fetlock joint in the same manner. A non-tiring tendinous supporting belt between the shoulder and elbow joints in the form of a powerful tendinous cord which passes through the biceps (Figure 8, d) also exists. It stretches in front of the shoulder joint and stops it from giving way when the elbow joint is locked. This supporting belt also extends a tendon branch (Figure 8, d') to the carpal joint, through which the belt remains under tension. The forward pull of the biceps is counterbalanced on the rear surface of the elbow joint by the thin and tendinous superficial and deep flexor muscles of the toe (superficial and deep digital flexor tendons, Figure 8, a and b). If this continuous tendon cord running from the rear surface of the humerus down to the toe is taut on the limb which is taking the weight, it also supports the elbow joint, preventing it from giving way. This enables the forelegs to stand without tiring.

During movement, the point of the elbow finds a delicate hold within a ring-shaped mass of strong muscles in which the position of the elbow and shoulder joints is counterbalanced to a certain extent. The angle of the shoulder blade and the position of the neck are in accordance to this counterbalance. A bundle of strong muscles, the extensors of the elbow (Figure 8, e), extends from the rear edge of the shoulder blade to the point of the elbow. Another muscle, the neck section of the lower serrated muscle (Figure 8, f), extends forward from the inner surface of the shoulder blade to the 7th to 4th cervical vertebra and pulls the upper part of the shoulder blade forward when the head is lowered or stretched. These same cervical vertebrae are finally anchored downward on the first rib by the scalene muscle (suspensory muscle of the ribs; Figure 8, g). Thus, when the neck is lowered, it exerts a pull on the point of the elbow by means of this ring of muscles and, as a direct consequence, stretches this joint whereby the shoulder is positioned at a steeper angle. Horses in which these muscles are strongly developed, frequently stand with their forelimbs camped out, even at rest, because the pull of the muscles positions the shoulder at a steeper angle. These muscles have only little tendinous reinforcement; together with the thoracic muscles, they are primarily movement muscles of the shoulder.

This extensive explanation of the static systems, which, at first, seem only to have been created for standing, was necessary to understand their function in movement. The mechanisms which are so practical for standing are responsible for the frequent tendon injuries in horses which have been over-worked. In this case, the tendinous ligament structures of the flexor tendons are primarily to blame. It must be emphasized again that these are supporting ligaments of the flexor tendons which belong to the flexor muscles. During movement in the supporting phase, the flexor tendons which support the overextension of the digital joints are held elastically on their muscles. When the muscles tire as a result of overexertion and, consequently, become painful, and if the tendons did not possess supporting ligaments, the horse would stop because of the pain. If the horse was nevertheless forced to continue to canter on, pulled muscles or even tears would appear as those observed in humans and also in the dog. The supporting ligaments, however, allow the horse to keep moving and to relax the painful muscles in the supporting phase. Henceforth, the taut tendinous supporting apparatus is no longer capable of taking the enormous strain and its fibers tear. Never has one of the flexor tendons above their supporting ligaments, e.g., between the supporting ligament and the muscle, been affected; proof that passive strain and not active muscle function is the cause of tendon injury.

The suspensory ligament and the superficial digital flexor tendon experience the greatest strain as the limbs support the weight of the body – therefore, especially during landing after a jump (passive strain), while the deep digital flexor tendon achieves maximum tension during the moment of pushing off from the ground (active strain). This also explains why the latter is very seldom injured, mostly in cart horses.

Strongly developed muscles on the forearm are characteristic in high-stamina hunting horses. It is not unreasonable to expect a great durability of the tendons of such horses; on the one hand, because the stronger muscles do not tire so quickly and, on the other hand, because their tendons have become more resistant through training.

The tendinous supporting belt of the shoulder joint is rarely affected by injury. This can be explained by its connection to the elbow joint, which is in a state of delicate counterbalance. This makes it impossible for the tendinous supporting belt to be used in a purely static function during movement.

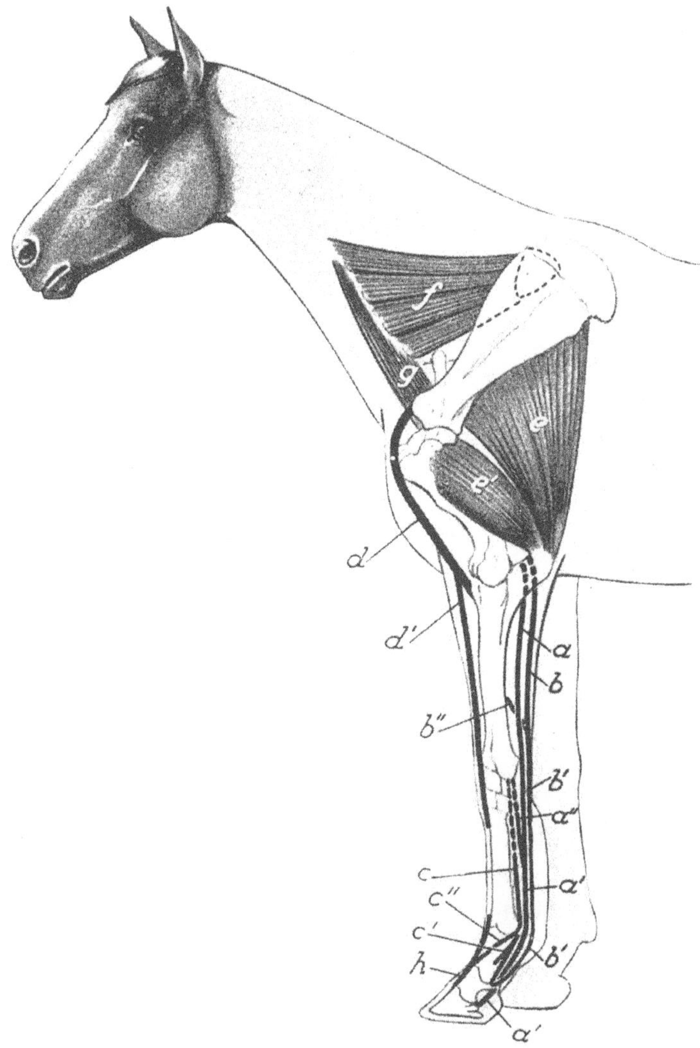

Figure 8: Die Muskeln des Schulterrings und die statischen Einrichtungen an der Vordergliedmaße des Pferdes in der linken Ansicht

- **a** Deep digital flexor muscle, *M. flexor digitalis profundus*
- **a'** Deep digital flexor muscle
- **a"** Supporting ligament
- **b** Superficial flexor muscle, *M. flexor digitalis superficialis*
- **b'** Superficial flexor muscle
- **b"** Supporting ligament
- **c, c', c"** Suspensory ligament, namely:
- **c** proximal (upper) sesamoideum boned ligaments (splint bone), *M. interosseus medius*
- **c'** distal (lower) sesamoideum boned ligament
- **c"** connection cord to digital extensor tendon
- **d** Biceps muscle of upper arm, *M. biceps brachii*
- **d'** Tendon branch to the carpal joint, *Lacertus fibrosus*
- **e, e'** Extensor of the elbow
- **f** The cervical part of the lower serrated muscle, *M. serratus ventralis cervicis*
- **g** The suspensory muscle of the ribs, *M. scalenus primae costae*
- **h** The common digital extensor tendon

b) The Forehand During Jumping

The muscles of the shoulder and the torso are subject to maximum stress during a jump and when riding in hilly terrain. Insufficient thrust from the hindquarters can be compensated by approaching the jump at greater speed; the length of the jump always depends on the speed of the approach; conversely, energetically pushing the forehand off from the ground is a contributory factor how high the horse jumps. As it lands, the horse's entire bodyweight falls on the forehand, which acts as a shock absorber, counterbalances, and immediately pushes off again. At first view, the horse does not seem to have any means of compensating or facilitating the situation. It is, however, the case. The degree to which the weight on the forehand is lightened depends on the technique during landing and on how experienced the horse is. Firstly, a comparison: If a person catches a heavy iron ball thrown to them in midair and tries to hold it with their arm extended, their arm will be sprained and the ball will slip out of their hand. If, however, this person draws their arm and whole body back in the same direction as the flight path of the ball in the instant when the ball touches their hand, cushioning the impact, then a person can catch incredibly heavy weights. A person's knee bend is another suitable example; stronger extensor muscles on the femur make it possible to absorb the impact of jumping off from a greater height. These comparisons are not entirely accurate, however, because a horse never jumps into a complete standstill but continues moving forward. The fact that the movement continues to flow during landing is the decisive factor. The inexperienced horse lands on a fully supporting front limb which takes on the entire body weight in that moment. The limb is extended in the course of this. The rider perceives this landing as a jolt: the flow of movement is interrupted for a fraction of a second; the horse literally has to collect itself to canter on. Such a landing is not part of harmonious forward movement (Figures 9 and 10); it compresses the forelimb and would cause injury more frequently if the limb was not elastically connected with the torso to cushion the impact (through the suspensory muscles of the torso). The loud groan which horses often make after an awkward landing is an indication of how unpleasant they find such bruising on the forehand. In some horses, one can simply induce this groan if one pulls the head of the horse up during landing and thus stops the transfer of the weight over the forehand.

An experienced jumper lands fluently (Figure 11). The foreleg which is set down first is not placed in the body's trajectory of landing, but a little behind it; the weight maintains its overload to the front, is only slowed down, and then taken by the other foreleg which has extended far forward to set down on the ground and supports the entire weight. The fetlock joint of this leg is often so strongly bent that the ergot touches the ground, while the other front leg is already bent and swung forward. The horse therefore supports itself with only one foreleg.

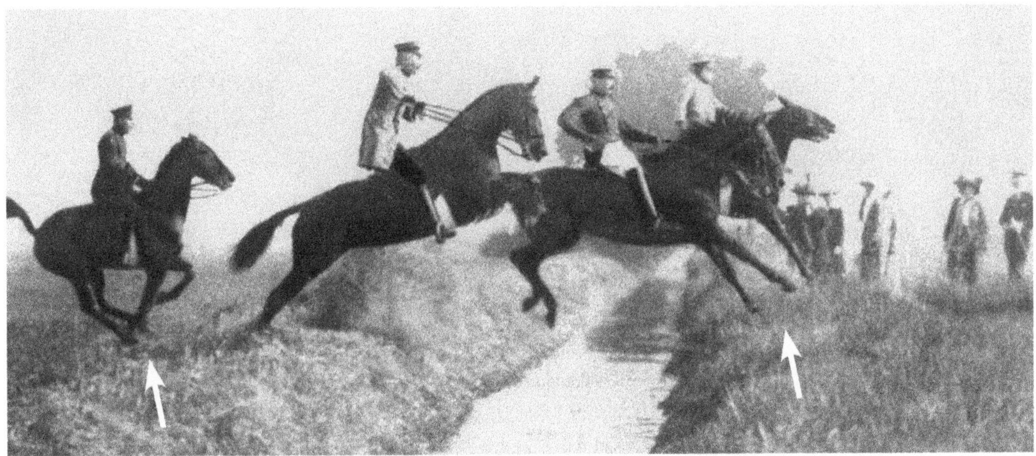

Figure 9: Both horses in the process of landing are obstructed in the mouth by their riders; they set down their forelegs in an extended position short of the point where they should land (trajectory) and will pull up sharply. The last horse (on the left) is already pushing off with its forelegs as the hindquarters are just set down.

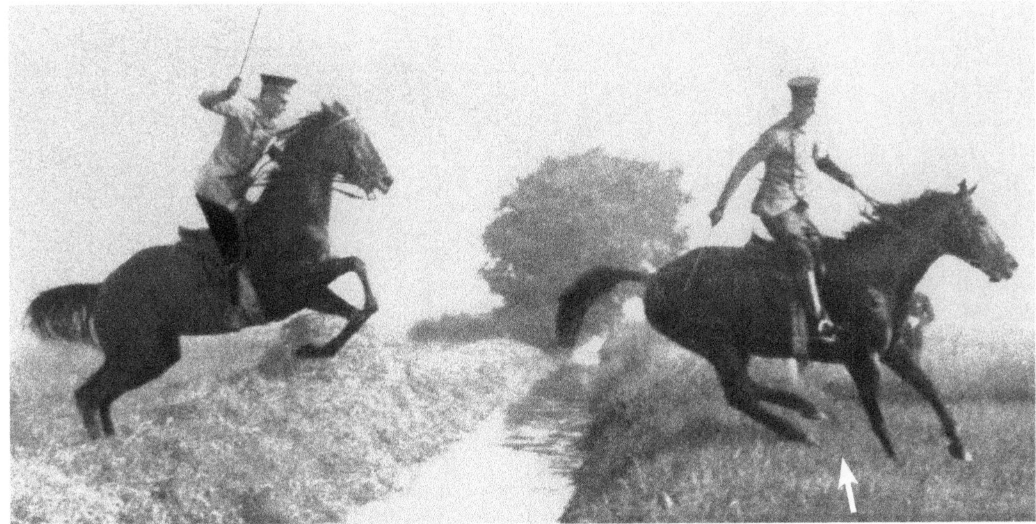

Figure 10: A horse is pulled up completely 'on all fours' during the landing. Horse and rider literally ram into the ground and stop moving forward completely. The rider is hanging onto the reins.

Only then is the hind leg set down. Next, the other supporting foreleg pushes off into a new canter stride. Some fast horses do this even before the hind legs have touched the ground (Figure 9, see above), proof that pushing off with the forehand is important for the jump itself and also to continue to canter on swiftly after the jump. Balancing the body over the forehand is imperative to retain the flow of the movement. To achieve this, the connecting muscles between the shoulder on the one side, and the neck, thoracic cage, and back on the other, are used. The connecting muscles to the neck act on the upper part of the shoulder

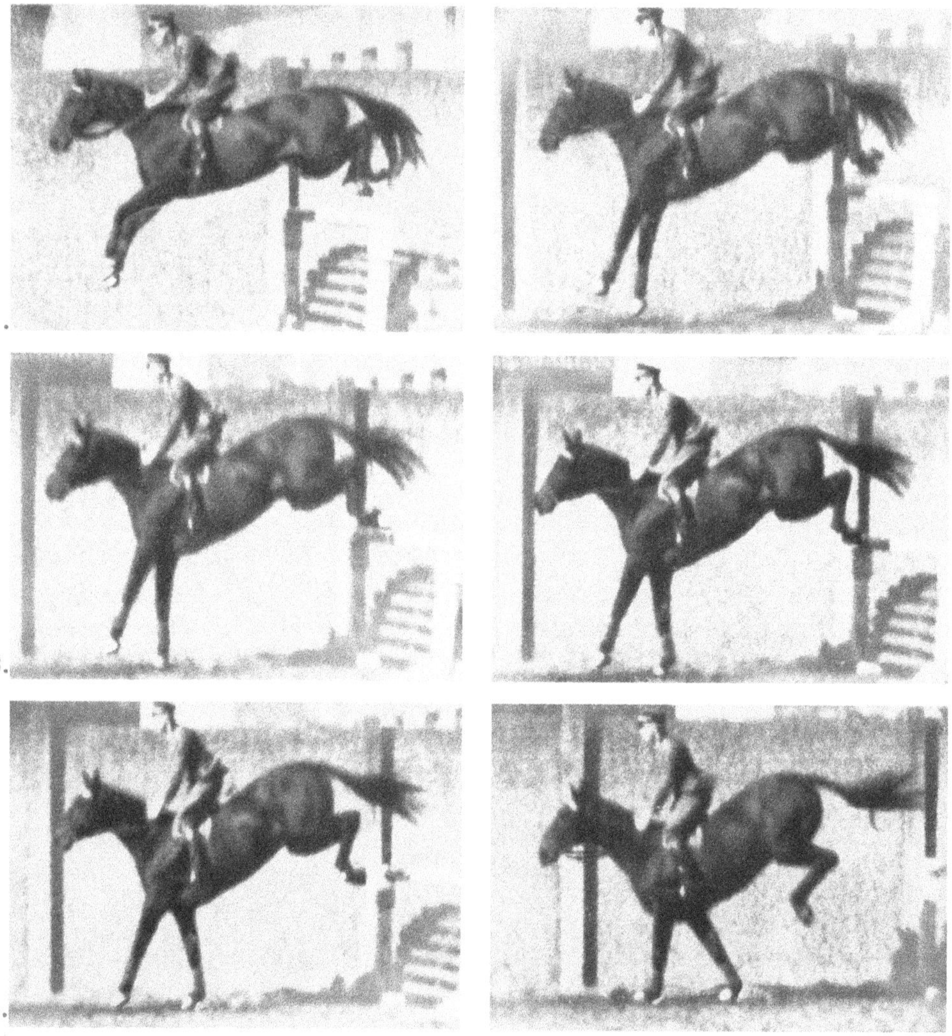

1. 2. 3. 4. 5. 6. 7.

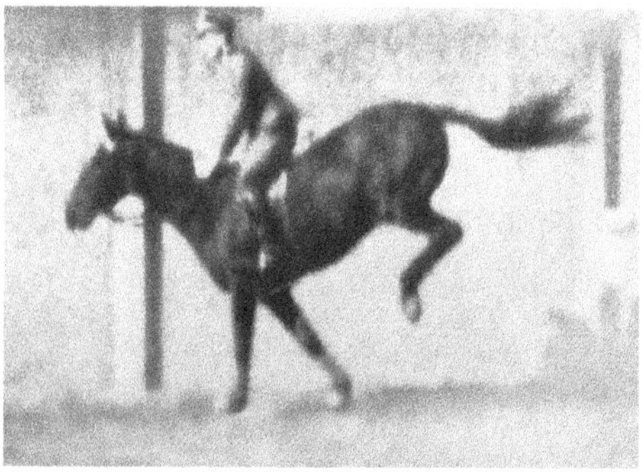

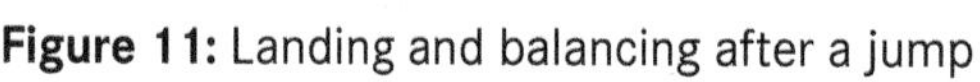

Figure 11: Landing and balancing after a jump

1. The right front leg is beginning to extend.
2. The right front leg is placed behind the trajectory of landing and reaches for the ground.
3. The right front leg is set down behind the trajectory of landing.

4./5. The right front leg slows down the descending body mass. The fetlock joint is only slightly bent, proof that this leg is not taking the whole weight. The main part of the weight rolls through the right leg onto the left front leg which is extended along the trajectory of the landing.

6. The left front leg begins to support and to take the weight.
7. The left front leg is supporting fully. The overextended fetlock is proof that it is taking the entire weight. The right front leg extends to lift off the ground.

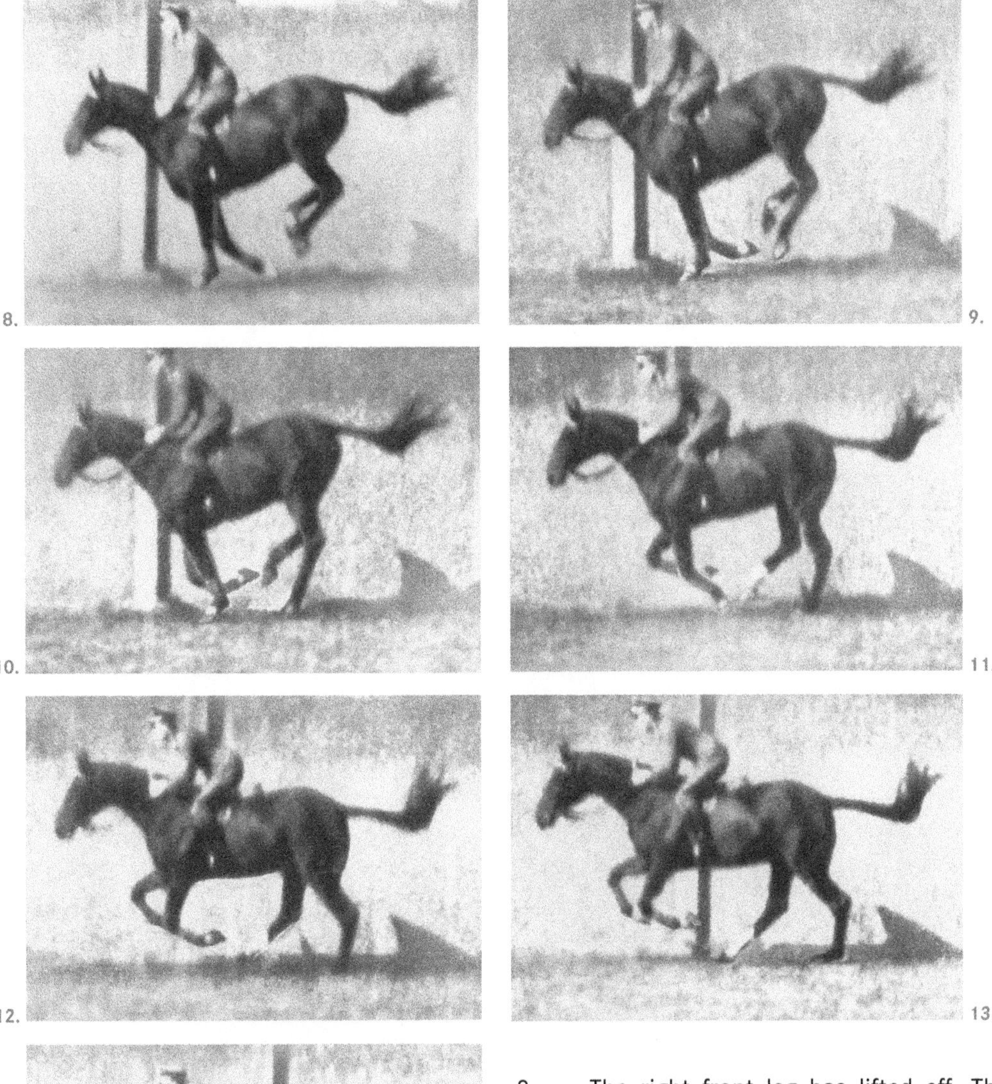

8.–10. The right front leg has lifted off. The left leg extends to lift off. The position of horse and rider clearly shows how the body is balancing over the left supporting front leg. The left hind leg sets down on the ground.

11. The left front leg pushes off before the right hind has made contact with the ground, the left hind leg is supporting.

12.–14. The horse lifts itself into an elevated canter stride only once the right hind leg has been set down on the ground and then develops to lift off out of the greatest possible angle (of flexion).

blade and the muscles which connect to the back and thoracic cage act on the lower part of the shoulder blade and the upper forearm. This is how the rotation of the shoulder blade during landing is elastically stabilized on the neck and torso, just as the unrestricted development of power of the forehand during take-off is dependent on the position of the neck and back.

Today it is generally recognized that horses should land with their necks stretched and not held high – a knowledge which has been gained through experiences in equestrian performance sports. The neck carriage is literally not a 'position' but rather a movement, an activity. The horse's neck stretches forward during landing, brings most of its body mass forward, allowing the weight to be transferred over the leg that was initially set down on the ground, which, as a result, is prevented from being put under too much stress. Simultaneously, the neck thus pulls taut the "spring" (the cervical section of the serrated muscle) between the cervical spine and the upper part of the shoulder and stabilizes it elastically. The neck is stretched to the maximum in the moment just before the horse pushes off. Now the connecting muscle to the shoulder can function with the greatest possible strength out of maximum extension and stretch the shoulder to push off. During this same phase, the extension of the upper neck muscles causes the back to arch (see Chapter 2) and the action of the broad back muscles (Figure 4, h, see Page 33) between the upper arm, back, and loins pulls the hind leg forward to be set down on the ground. The neck is raised again just before the hindquarters touch the ground. In the process, the effect of the muscle swinging the foreleg forward (head-neck-arm muscle, Figure 4, i) is shifted toward the head, and the foreleg can reach further forward.

How important it is for a horse to stretch its neck forward to balance can best be observed by how it jumps onto a high bank. Often, it almost touches the ground with its nose, the hand of the rider follows the head far forward or lets the reins slip. If the rider impedes the action of the neck, the horse is at best impaired in its movement and stops on the bank; but if the rider hangs onto the reins, the horse can even fall backwards (Figures 12 and 13).

c) Movement and Training of the Forehand

The movement of the forehand is divided into four phases; swinging forward, setting down, supporting, and swinging off the ground. It is unnecessary to go into greater detail as the rider is only interested in the elasticity and scope of the movement. Riders want to understand the cause of a dull and short movement of healthy horses. In the preceding chapters it has already been pointed out that the movement of the foreleg is dependent on the carriage of the neck, the action of the back, and the natural movement of the hind legs. This complex interdependence explains why there are no gymnastic exercises specifically for the forehand that can be carried out in the arena, as opposed to those for the hindquarters. The movement of the forehand develops of its own accord if the action of the back, hindquarters, and the position of the neck are correct. If the movement of the hind legs is abnormally stiff or straight, the weight of the body falls more onto the forehand, the movement becomes dull, the front legs remain planted on the ground for too long and do not push off with enough impulsion. The weight of the body is more or less sluggishly transferred from one front leg to the other. If the back has become stiff due to incorrect use of its muscles, the broad back muscle (Figure 4, h, see Page 33), which extends from the loins to the upper arm, is simultaneously tightened and, thus, the front leg stepping forward is restricted. The horse's steps and strides are inevitably shortened. The head-neck-arm muscle (Figure 4, i) which, as its name suggests, runs from the head and neck to the upper arm, swings the front leg forward. This muscle is responsible for the scope of the horse's movement by controlling the position of the neck. In racehorses where the neck is stretched far forward but straight, the action of the forehand is flat and extended, but when the neck is raised higher, the forehand action is high and does not cover much ground (knee action, carpal joint). A foreshortened neck, (whether by being contracted in the form of an ewe neck or by the horse coming to low and behind the vertical), shortens the range of action of the head-neck-arm muscle and, thus, the range of the foreleg. Only when the rider attains the perfect neck carriage, which combines maximum stretch of the neck with the relative raise of the forehand, can the horse develop an elevated and ground-covering movement.

Therefore, the movement of the forehand is of secondary importance within the framework of a horse's overall training process. This is quite a different matter in the daily training, which only a few riders fully comprehend.

It is a widely held misconception that the hindquarters should be made to step further underneath the horse's body to take weight off the "more delicate" forehand. In the past, this concept led to riders having to sit as far back as possible in the saddle and even forcing the horse to land on the hindquarters after a jump. This concept confused cause and effect. It is not by taking weight off it that we can create and maintain a strong and healthy forehand, but a suitable training must focus on strengthening and encouraging the growth of the muscles in the forearm and shoulder which **automatically makes the tendons more resilient.** Of course, by means of gymnastic work in the outdoor arena, in combination with frequent jumping over obstacles, appropriate to the particular level of

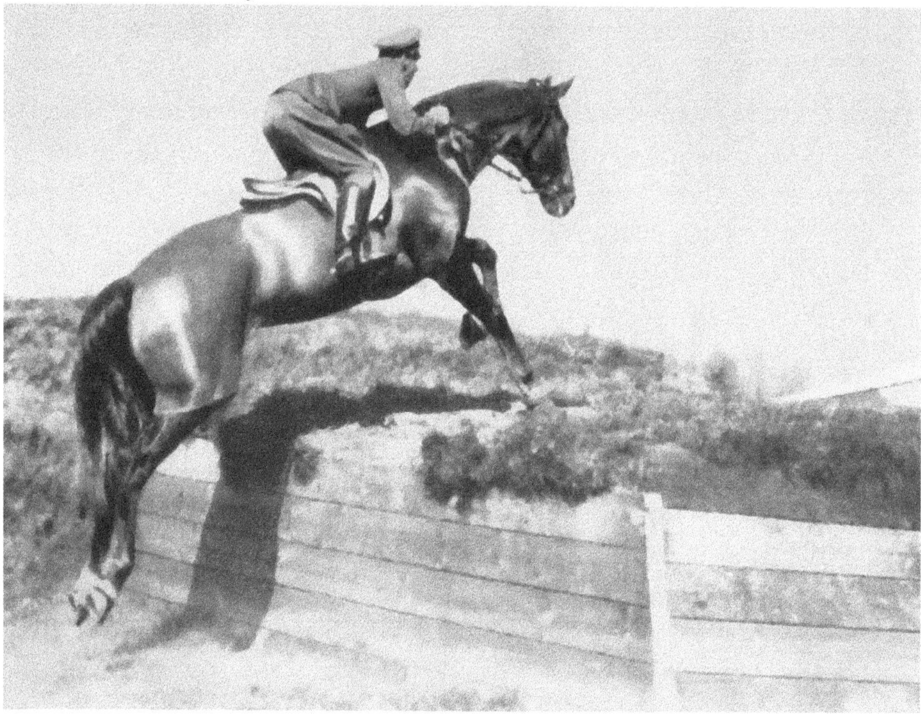

Figure 12: Jumping onto the bank in an exemplary, supple position

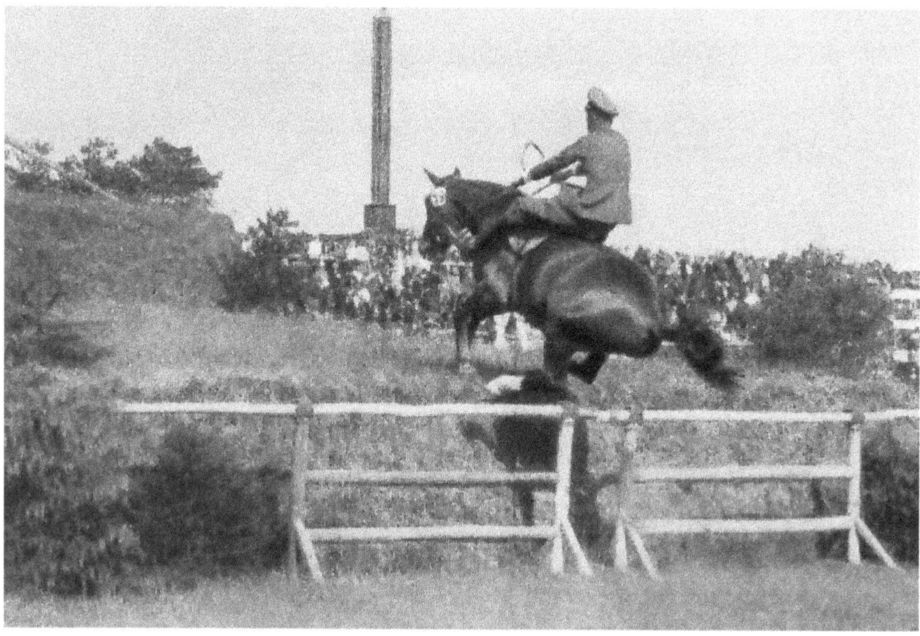

Figure 13: Jumping onto the bank. The rider is behind the movement and hangs onto the reins. By strongly buckling in the knees, the horse is trying to bring its center of gravity forward and just manages to step on the edge of the bank with its hind legs.

training of the horse, one can improve the elasticity of the ligaments and tendons – and many indestructibly tough horses have only had this type of training. However, if we look at the general principle, this type of work really starts at the wrong point. Whereas during correct riding on the flat, the muscles of the forehand are never overworked to the point of extreme fatigue as compared to the hindquarters, we expect these muscles of the forehand to absorb the entire body weight during landing after a jump – meaning the highest level of strain in the sense of stretching these muscles. If the muscles lack the absolute strength needed to maintain the necessary tension for this, they will be overextended as they relax and the superficial digital flexor tendon, together with its supporting check ligaments, and the suspensory ligament of the fetlock will carry the entire weight and become injured. Hence, developing muscular strength must be the primary aim of training, as it is just as important for the forehand as is generally emphasized for the hindquarters. Once again, it is the most natural gait of the horse, the canter, which achieves this goal: however, not periods of 1 to 2 minutes in the arena but rather a long, quiet canter over a distance across country. One does need to be a very skillful rider to make even the youngest horses canter at an even pace after they have understood that this is not a rare and exciting excuse to 'let rip', but rather that they will frequently be required to canter to the point of exhaustion. Fatigue substances (lactic acid) in the muscles are the best growth stimulant, provided that they remain at levels at which the circulation of the blood is not adversely affected. Overexertion goes in tandem with swelling of the muscles as a result of accumulation of fatigue substances and is harmful. Long, steady rides practically never result in overexertion as opposed to the extreme demands caused by high speed or very deep footing. It is not difficult for a rider who knows their horse to learn to judge how tired the horse is. Apart from the general impression, other palpable and visible indications of tiredness are tripping in walk, the fetlock occasionally knuckling over until the ergot touches the ground, and a lack of stability in the carpal joint. The lack of stability in the carpal joint is often erroneously perceived as a fault or weakness in a tired but otherwise healthy horse. Quite the opposite is the case: This position takes the strain off the tendons below their supporting ligaments and makes the muscles work; tendon injuries are rare in such horses.

If a young horse is used to long distances and has also received general dressage training, it will start training over fences with more body strength and more consideration. Where available, rough and hilly terrain, in which both the forehand and hindquarters will be thoroughly gymnastically trained, should be used extensively.

In conclusion, the following are necessary for the training and muscular development of the forehand: quiet canter work over considerably long distances at a natural pace (a steady canter), riding on uneven terrain, and climbing promote muscle growth without the danger of overtaxing the forehand and provide the horse with the strength required later for maximum levels of performance at speed or jumping. Whether these principles are applicable in the training of young thoroughbreds in racing can only be tested in practice– a worthwhile and perhaps profitable undertaking.

6

The Abdominal Muscles

a) Notes on Anatomical Function (Figure 4, see Page 33)

The abdominal muscles are primarily intended to carry the contents of the abdominal cavity. In their secondary role, they are muscles of movement. The transverse abdominal and oblique internal abdominal muscle suspend the abdomen and thorax, together with their contents, like a "hammock" on the loins and the coxal tuberosity. The principal role of the rectus (straight) abdominal muscle (Figure 4, t) is (together with the strong fascia of the abdominal walls) also that of a "hammock" as well as acting as a static organ for the lower brace of the vertebral bridge between the sternum and pelvis (see Chapter 2). The longitudinal muscles on both sides meet in the middle in the white line, a coarse tendinous anatomical structure. In its contracted state, the straight abdominal muscle can pull the lower edge of the pelvis forward, thereby arching the back upward and allowing the hind leg to swing far underneath the horse's body. The muscle is divided into sections by transverse tendinous strips; this increase in work force also increases the muscle's strength. The oblique external abdominal muscle (Figure 4, u) originates on the outside of the ribs in an ascending line from the elbow almost to the coxal tuberosity. Next to this muscle's attachment by its end-tendons on the white line and the pelvis, the rider is mostly interested in the fact that it extends onto the inner surface of the femurs with its broad tendinous sheet and, together with the *Musculus cutaneous trunci* (abdominal skin muscle), forms their fascia covering. In this manner, the muscle plays a part in the movement of the hind leg.

b) The Function of the Abdominal Muscles

The function of carrying the viscera need not be taken into consideration here. There is a general tendency to attach too much importance to the abdominal muscles as muscles of movement. Their dual function and the course over which they extend in an arch across the curved surface of the abdomen eliminate a large development of power between the thorax and the pelvis. Constant contraction of these muscles would exert an unbearable pressure on the intestines of the horse and also inhibit breathing as a result of their partial origin on the mobile costal (rib) arch. The previously taught concept that the pelvis was pulled forward with flexion in the sacroiliac joint during "collection" would mean that the horse would permanently contract the abdominal muscles whereby the horse's breathing would be impeded. The abdominal muscles come into play as muscles of movement during canter by swinging the hindquarters forward and under in the moment of suspension, when they do not have to overcome a lot of resistance. The pull of the straight abdominal muscle on the pelvis does not solely affect the flexion of the sacroiliac joint, but also flexes the entire back upward in a convex elastic arch. The back comes up under the seat of the rider. The rider can tell by the horse's breathing that the oblique external abdominal muscle, which connects the costal (rib) arch with the inner surface of the femur, only functions rhythmically in the canter. While breathing is not uniformly related to the rhythm of the movement in walk and trot, all horses breathe in the rhythm of the canter. They inhale as the hind legs swing forward and exhale during pushing off from the ground.

According to an old farmers' tale, mares in foal should walk and trot in harness, but they should not be ridden. The deeper meaning for this rule is both the increased concussion and the hard work required of the abdominal muscles in canter. It is also rarely possible to re-form a so-called potbelly, whether it is a grass belly or a result of being in foal, by working in harness, while young horses will regain their slim shape within six months to a year if worked consistently in canter. The slack abdominal muscles are thereby strengthened and become taut and toned again.

The oblique external abdominal muscle and abdominal skin muscle will be referred to again in the section on leg aids. It is sufficient to mention here that the use of the leg aid or spur on one side causes a reflex contraction of these muscles which effects the inner surface of the femur. As these muscles are strong enough to pull the hind leg on the same side forward, the reflex only gives the impulse to initiate the movement. The horse must learn to interpret this aid correctly and to follow the reaction which has been caused by it.

7

The Aids

[Paul] Plinzner [and Gustav Steinbrecht in *The Gymnasium of the Horse*, Xenophon Press 1994] needs 30 pages in his book [*Gymnasium of the Horse*, Xenophon Press 1994] on the gymnastic training of the horse just to explain the general principles of the aids, in addition to the specific way to take influence in the various movements. This appears too difficult for the average rider; they will most likely not be able to understand how their aids influence the horse's body by studying such equestrian literature. But this is essential if the rider is to use the aids correctly.

There are driving and regulating aids. Used evenly on both sides they act in a straight direction, if applied only on one side, they act sideways. The straight direction is the most natural for the horse and it must therefore first learn to react positively to these aids. If the rider starts riding curved lines too early or even introduces leg-yield, the horse will be more likely to resist, which initially manifests itself in an uneven step sequence.

a) The Driving Leg Aid

should be the principal and always dominant aid. It is said with good reason that a horse must always be on the rider's leg. The influence which the rider is capable of achieving by using their **lower leg** are the most natural and effective. The pressure of the rider's leg acts on the hind leg on the same side by means of the muscles situated there. The oblique external abdominal muscle of the horse originates on the ribs and, in conjunction with the abdominal skin muscle, covers the sides of the abdominal wall. Hence, both muscles are situated where the rider's leg touches and exert a pull on the inner surface of the femur and stifle respectively. Stimulating these muscles by pressure from the leg or use of the spur causes them to contract, which results in the horse bringing its femur forward and bending the hip joint. If this reaction were independent of the horse's will, we could say that activating the hindquarters and, ultimately, collection would be a purely mechanical matter.

However, it is not that simple. The use of the leg or spur always produces an active reaction in the young horse, but in the form of twitching the skin as a defensive movement against the touch as in the case of a fly bite. Often, the respective hind leg is brought forward to be able to move the skin more. The horse must learn to correctly interpret the reflex initiated by the leg aid and to listen to it by lifting, flexing, and stepping forward with the hind foot. It is a long process before this is achieved. It begins by applying very strong pressure evenly on both sides with the rider's legs, whereby the entire length of the rider's lower leg must lie flat against the horse. The young horse perceives this pressure merely as duress but does not know how to react to it. This is why it must be immediately followed with a touch of the whip. As soon as the horse moves forward, the pressure is significantly reduced, however, the contact of the leg on the horse must not be lost. Soon the horse will not wait for the whip aid but go forward at the pressure of the leg because it knows that this pressure, which it finds unpleasant, will then be reduced. If the pressure of the leg is increased during movement, the horse will move faster. This desired effect must be consistently followed by relieving the horse by means of a significant reduction in the pressure of the leg which is then applied steadily again. These aids must be very fine-tuned; the stronger leg aid must never be used surprisingly for the horse. The horse must always first prick its ears attentively and then allow itself to be pushed forward almost hesitantly. It must always accept the driving aids in any gait, i.e., it must willingly lengthen its steps and strides as a result of increased pressure from the leg, maintain a regular speed on steady, even pressure, and, when the pressure is taken off, either make a transition into the next lower gait or come to a halt. This requires the rider to be able to sit quietly and always maintain a driving contact with the lower leg, which should lie against the side of the rib cage without pronounced pressure. One can only control the rhythmic movement by use of the driving aid; the regulating aid, which will be discussed later, plays a minor role in this.

Thus far, the driving leg aid has only been described in the context of forward movement. In conjunction with a half-halt, it serves to collect the horse. The leg aid applied on one side or rather alternately should make the hind legs alternately flex and step further underneath the horse's body. It has nothing to do with the sideways driving aid. Before we move on to this, we must visualize the torso action of the horse during movement. If a horse is led away from us in walk, we can observe that the torso swings from side to side with every step. These swinging movements are nothing more than a balancing of the weight within the "mass of the horse." If, for example, the right hind leg steps forward, the left supporting leg takes the entire weight; this therefore swings over to the left so that it remains supported in a vertical position. These movements become even more exaggerated in a horse which lets its back sag, the longer the stride becomes. In correctly ridden horses, movements of the tail are the only indication of these swinging movements, but they are present and the rider can feel them.

The rider to whom these facts are new should let their lower legs hang completely free (dangling) in walk. The rider will then notice that these swing in the rhythm of the movement on alternate sides against the horse's body, and also make contact with it. The lower leg of the rider following the swinging movement of the horse's torso falls against the side of the rib cage in the same moment as the swinging motion stops and the hind leg on the same side sets down on the ground. If the leg aid is given in this sequence of legs, producing the reflex action of the lateral abdominal muscles as described above and the horse reacts correctly, then the hip joint will be flexed as the limb is placed on the ground and this initiates the flexion of the haunches. Phlegmatic horses need a strong alternating leg aid and, very often, one cannot avoid using the spur. There are excellent and highly successful dressage riders who use these alternate leg aids so obviously that they are clearly visible to the spectator. The ideal, however, is to refine giving the aids in dressage so that it becomes invisible to the spectator. In principle, the lower leg lying evenly against the horse carries out this very function. With every step or stride, the horse automatically receives the unilateral aid from the leg or spur lying against its side, as in the moment when the foot is set down, the pressure of the rider's leg must act more strongly on this side (as explained above), because the sideways swinging movement stops and the wall of the rib cage now comes toward the leg.

In this respect it must be stressed that a horse resents nothing as much as excessive flexion in the haunches elicited by unfeeling and harsh use of the rein aids which do not permit it to come out of this flexed gait (see Chapter 4). The horse then fights with all the means at its disposal to escape this strenuous gymnastic exercise and learns to do exactly the opposite by consciously suppressing the reflex of the abdominal muscles of the sides, i.e., it becomes dead to the leg. The same effect is achieved by insensitive active use of the leg which bears no relation to the speed or sequence of legs. Simultaneously, a flapping leg on the part of the rider is a mistake which is frequently seen. Old school horses accept it stoically, without reacting to it, while horses which are correctly ridden and obedient to the leg become nervous because they do not know how to respond to this "aid."

There is nothing to be added here beyond the "principles of riding" on how to use the sideways driving leg aid, the canter aid, and all the other movements.

b) The Regulating Aid, Thoroughness, and Problems Which May Arise

Rein aids as a regulating aid can only be described as an **aid** in the truest sense of the word if the horse is on the driving aids. Otherwise, it is at best a means of braking and steering, depending on the horse's temperament, except if used with an inconsiderate level of abusive force.

The basis for the influence of the rein is constant contact on the bit. Contact is most important and attainable for all horses. Only when contact is established can carriage gradually be developed, which must vary according to each individual horse. It is not only dependent on the shape of the neck and the throat latch, but also on the conformation of the body as a whole, especially of the back and hindquarters.

In contact, the bit rests calmly and evenly on the bars of the mouth and the tongue. The mouthpiece of the snaffle is supported mostly on the bars of the mouth as a result of its middle joint; the horse holds the mouthpiece of a double bridle without a port in a straight position flat on the tongue; with a little port, it just touches the bars of the mouth; with a larger port, the bit rests on the bars. The strong effect of the double bridle is caused by the lever action of the curb chain and cheek bars (shanks), which, together, exert a pressure on the bars of the horse's mouth which no rider's hand could achieve with a snaffle with the same intensity.

We differentiate between a light and strong contact, depending on whether the horse lightly rests the bars of its mouth against the mouthpiece of the bit and takes the reins evenly or whether it leans on the bit and pulls heavily on the reins. Only a light and steady contact leads to the desired aim: throughness and, later, carriage of the horse.

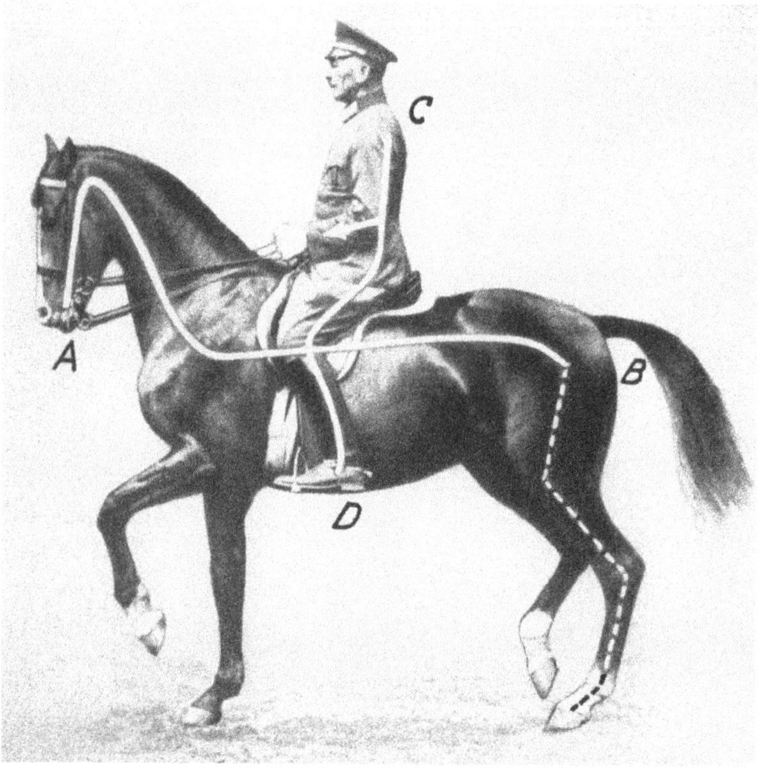

Figure 14: Schematic diagram representing the lines of force along which the aids take an effect on the horse's body.

Throughness simply means that the asking rein aid, the half-halt, takes effect through the horse's whole body and flexes the joints of the hind limbs.

Let us imagine a horse whose carriage was absolutely stable from the bars of its mouth right through to the croup. In such a horse, the white line A to B shown in Figure 14 would be inflexible. The half-halt would then have to act on the joints of the hind legs, making the horse creep backward if the forward driving leg aid was missing. But if the leg simultaneously activates the hindquarters to step forward and under, the horse would have no alternative but to flex the joints of its hindquarters. Let us furthermore imagine that the seat of the rider is similarly solid and that the line C to D in the same drawing always has the same inclination angle to the line A to B. If the line C to D even slightly inclined toward the back, it would have a corresponding effect on the line A to B and thereby produce flexion in the joints of the hindquarters, i.e., a rotation of the intersection of the lines A to B and C to D with simultaneous lowering of the croup and elevation of the forehand. However, both these lines are not fixed on a living horse but flexible like elastic rods. If they were solidly fixed, the hindquarters could be flexed by using force. Yet, the elasticity of these lines demands a fine coordination of the effect of the aids and the forces at play. On the other hand, this elasticity facilitates the seamless transitions which we so admire in a horse which is ridden perfectly. Herein lies the secret of the so-called "good hand," to always keep this elastic bow in an almost constant state of tension, never to overdraw and let it become tight, but never to completely release the tension. In other words, the contact, the weight that the reins place in the rider's hands, should always remain as constant as possible. But only the rider who has the hindquarters on their driving aids can work with this elastic bow. Only then can the most delicate half-halt work through the entire horse. Otherwise, the bow is only spanned from the hand through the neck to the bars of the mouth and the reins back to the hand; the horse becomes tight in the neck and the half-halt is stuck with the rider. Or the horse resists the stronger rein aid and evades it in an upward direction. For practical riding, it should be deduced from these theoretical concepts that the half-halt on a school horse does not mean shortening the reins and then pulling but shifting the weight through a short, just perceptible straightening of the rider's body. The rider does not need to bend their arm. This would be the ideal which is neither attainable for all horses nor for all riders.

Without doubt, the most difficult hurdle during training is teaching a horse throughness. When searching for the reason, one must start with the hindquarters. The flexed gait is physically demanding; as the horse becomes increasingly tired it certainly experiences muscle pains. If the rider continued to ask too much of the horse and it remained through, the muscle pains would continue to increase; as a result, the horse would literally punish itself with every step because it is through. If, however, it stretches the joints of the hindquarters and gives up throughness, these muscles can rest. The horse learns very quickly through experience that resisting the rein aids of the rider is much more comfortable and less strenuous than the flexed gait which is required of it. It gets used to an incorrect carriage which we generally describe as dental problems or problems in the throat latch, neck, back, and movement. Whichever of these difficulties predominate, the horse always achieves the same: namely that the half-halt does not go through all the way to the hindquarters, it simply "gets stuck."

Having identified the hindquarters as the source of all our problems and perceived that everything else is of secondary importance, we should on no account attach less importance to these secondary problems. Only through a thorough knowledge of the long path which a half-halt must follow can riders who are still lacking the most sensitive feel find out where the half-halt gets stuck, how the horse deals with it, and what corrective measures are available.

Dental issues. Every rider should carefully feel the bars of the mouths of 100 horses, after having looked at an anatomical specimen of the bones of the lower jaw. This rider would then realise that there are bars with sharp edges and completely rounded bars. Sharp-edged bars are, of course, much more sensitive than round ones; they require a thick light bit and a soft hand of the rider. Pressure points occur very easily on sharp bars on which the periosteum (tissue layer covering the bone) frequently becomes inflamed and very painful. It is not uncommon for new bone matter to form in the place where the bit rests during the course of the *periostitis* (inflammation of the membranous tissue covering of the bone), similar to an *exostosis* (bone spur; benign growth on the surface of a bone). This is how sharp bars can become blunt. It is self-evident that these horses display dental issues during this transformation; an inspection of the bars of their horse's mouths would spare the frustration of some riders. This also includes the knowledge that young mares sometimes have little canine teeth which do not have roots in the jawbone as in male horses, but perch more or less loosely in the gums. The surrounding area of these teeth is often inflamed and tender. These teeth are uncomfortable; they should be properly extracted. Sharp or diseased bars of the mouth can certainly be the cause of dental issues.

If the bars of the mouth are healthy, the pressure of the bit is not painful. If the horse refuses the contact, it does so purely to avoid flexing its haunches. Horses have only two methods of doing so. Either they lean on the bit and take away the rider's rein aids while pushing off the ground with almost straight hind legs and avoiding the supporting phase of flexing the haunches. Or they do not let the bit rest on the bars of the mouth, escape backward by suddenly bending very strongly in the throat latch, come "behind the bit," or they lift their head and let the bit slide from the bars against the molars; they are then above the bit. In these cases, they display a limited movement and take short, hurried or long, dragging steps to avoid a clearly defined phase of flexing. One then often hears the bit rattle, grinding of the teeth, or rhythmic chewing all of which always indicates unwillingness. The tongue often lies over the bit or even hangs out of the corner of the mouth. The reason why it is so difficult for many riders to correct such horses is because they cannot feel the rhythm and, therefore, cannot maintain it with their driving aids. Any correction that begins with an attempt to have an influence on the mouth will fail because it confuses cause and effect. First and foremost, the free natural movement must be restored, if necessary, by forgoing any contact. This can best be achieved in walk and canter. Once the rhythm has been restored and the horse allows itself to be ridden forward, the skillful rider does not need to do anything more than maintain an even, very light contact without worrying about the head-neck-carriage and follow all the horse's evasive movements so that it never succeeds in avoiding the bit. If the rider forces the horse to go forward rhythmically and purposefully with their driving aids, then the horse soon gives up the struggle. If the contact remains so light that the natural movement is not disturbed, the carriage of the horse under the rider will come of its own accord with the development of the movement and muscular strength.

It is much more difficult to correct horses which are heavy in the hand. The only remedy is to strengthen the hindquarters with consistent gymnastic work during which the forehand becomes gradually and relatively raised. Horses with this vice clench their molars together; they are "dead in the mouth." In fact, only with clenched teeth can they use the sternomandibular muscle, which runs from the sternum to the rear edge of the lower jaw, to bend the head down so strongly. The first thing to do is to make the horse chew the bit, have it accept the forward-driving aids, and become somewhat lazy. Shortened movement, half-halts, riding on the circle and in flexion, with frequent changes, and, ultimately, also skillfully riding with one rein are the suitable methods to correct this problem.

Now that the mistakes have been discussed, it is easy to understand **good contact and throughness**. The horse thereby holds the bit with its masticatory chewing muscles (muscles used for chewing), which means that, while the aperture of the lips is closed, the lower jaw is slightly open. The relaxed muscles of mastication do not make regular chewing movements but maintain the contact between the bars of the mouth and the bit by constantly moving it. This movement of the mouth turns the horse's saliva to foam, visible on the aperture of the lips. This yielding freedom of movement enables the rider to transmit smooth rein aids. One can compare the activity of the masticatory muscle with the technical term of a clutch. This freedom of movement must never be stopped by bridles or nosebands which are too tight; these should only stop the masticatory muscle becoming totally slack and the mouth opening wide.

We must also refer to another **major error in the use of the reins**. Many riders shorten the inside rein in a turn and do not give accordingly with the outside rein.

This [incorrectly shortened inside] rein now acts most strongly on the bend of the longitudinal axis of the horse, and this is why the horse tends to avoid this pressure by moving its lower jaw toward the inside. In the process, the whole head is often held in a crooked position; the rider sees the inside ear as being higher than the outside one. One calls this vice "tilting in the poll." The outside rein should maintain the contact in a turn, it should even be leading when riding in flexion. Therefore, the outside hand should go forward and give just as much as the inside hand asks for flexion. Only then can the contact in flexion, which should be the result of the bend along the longitudinal axis of the whole horse, remain even.

There is a good tool to give the beginner the feeling of even contact. One should wrap the separated reins around a short riding whip, so that they are of equal length and about 30 cm apart. The hands hold the reins between the middle and ring fingers, and the whip with the thumbs on top in a "roof-like" position. The whip, whose midpoint must remain above the crest, then shows exactly by how much the outside hand should go forward and the inside hand back to maintain an even contact, because one of the reins will flap as soon as a mistake is made with the hand. For this purpose, a well-ridden schoolmaster is essential. At the same time, this exercise will demonstrate to the rider that bend cannot be achieved solely by rein aids but rather that the leg and seat aids play the defining role.

Problems in the throat latch. This area is the space between the rear upper edge of the mandibular ramus of the lower jawbone and the cervical spine, respectively the muscles which lie beneath it. People frequently describe this area as being narrow and thick, but this is very rarely the case. This only occurs if the parotid gland, which is situated in this area, is very strongly developed and if the two mandibular rami are so close together that pressure is exerted on the parotid gland when the head is bent down. In this case, the parotid gland becomes clearly visible. A pudgy and very fleshy throat latch can certainly cause carriage problems in the horse's elevation but does not impede the horse stretching its neck or affect the contact. With correct training, these muscles have diminished by the time the horse achieves a relative raise of the forehand (elevation). The root cause of a thick and narrow throat latch is nearly always the horse's refusal to flex its haunches and disappears as the horse accepts the contact.

Neck problems are usually secondary, i.e., the horse makes all sorts of neck movements to avoid the bit because it does not want to be through. Primary neck problems only exist with badly developed upper neck muscles which must be strengthened through appropriate training (see Chapter 2). We will only mention here that horses with long, possibly even thin necks require the rider to have an extremely sensitive hand. With good reason, this type of neck is called "a dangerous neck". The very size of the bow, as described previously, entails that the effect of the reins is very strong, more so because these horses naturally offer good carriage.

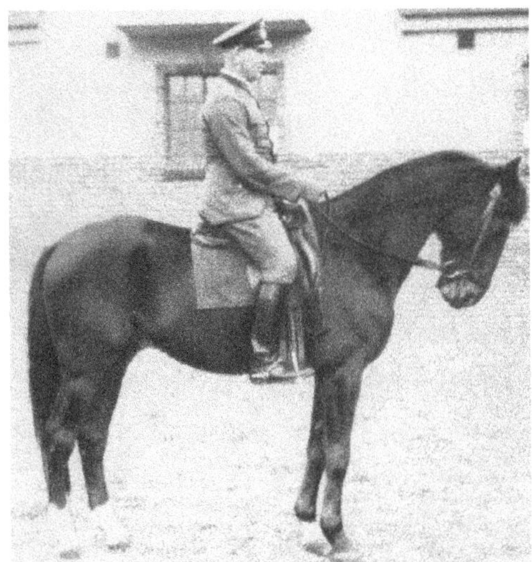

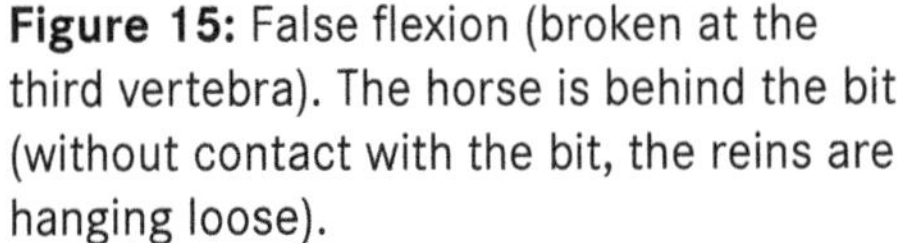

Figure 15: False flexion (broken at the third vertebra). The horse is behind the bit (without contact with the bit, the reins are hanging loose).

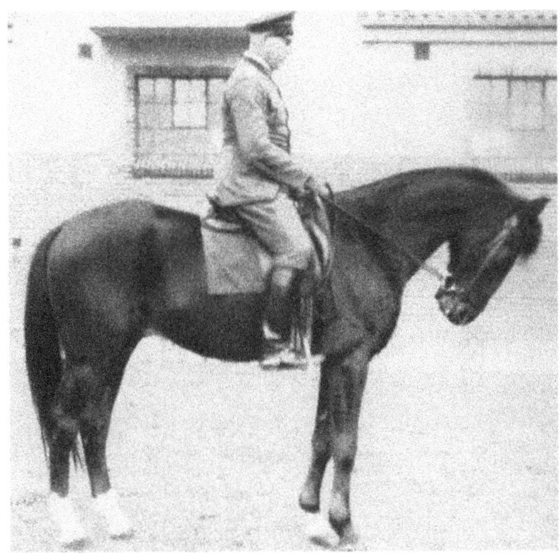

Figure 16: False flexion. The horse is leaning on the bit.

If the rider is tempted into working such horses faster, the hindquarters will easily be overworked and injuries will occur. Or the horse will develop neck problems, it will become tight in the neck and develop a "false bend." In the latter case, the horse bends its head strongly downward while keeping the neck raised. It achieves this with a muscle which extends from the 6th to 3rd (2nd) vertebra of the neck to the base of the skull, the deep flexor muscle of the head. The result is a bend that occurs between the 2nd and 3rd vertebra whereby the large crest of the 2nd vertebra of the neck makes the crest of the mane bulge upwards. Horses with this false bend are generally unpredictable with regard to contact; sometimes they are behind the bit, sometimes they lean on the bit but also accept the contact well (Figures 15 and 16). They use the false bend as a valve in which the rein aid gets stuck or not, as the horse wants. For the good rider, who has the horse on the driving aids, the false bend is not an impossible problem to correct.

Back problems. In addition to the methods of resisting the rein aids described in Chapters 2 and 3, we only have to mention hollowing and excessively arching the back, the so-called tensing of the back, as the horse can also evade throughness by this method. In doing so, the hind legs remain as straight as possible.

From these explanations, it becomes clear that throughness is the primary purpose of contact and of the rein aids, and that more or less perfect carriage can only be developed with thoroughness. Only the effective combination of driving and regulating aids leads to this goal.

c) The Interplay of the Aids

The most common mistake made by riders, which is the obsession to try to make the horse "carry itself" by means of various manipulations with their hands, will be mentioned first. By "see-sawing" – pulling the bit from side to side in the mouth or by frequently taking and giving the rein – they want to make the horse give in the throat latch and get it used to this carriage by constantly moving hands. By doing this, the riders merely work on the bars of the mouth and can also achieve a certain carriage as long as throughness is not required of the horse. With this method, one can also enter into a compromise with the horse so that it halts when the rider pulls more strongly on the reins as if on a verbal command. However, the observer can see that the transition to halt is abrupt, that the horse does not halt smoothly but simply comes to a halt by stopping with the forehand. If the rider is not careful, they fall forward as a result. But if something happens which makes the halt appear undesirable to such a horse, whether it is an extended canter or even while out hunting, it takes the rider's hand in either an upward or downward direction; the rider then pulls helplessly on the reins and has no further influence on the speed. Thus, this more or less skillful fiddling about with the bit can only result in a round neck position. Everything behind the saddle – the back and hindquarters – remain not only unaffected, but the natural sequence of the movement is disturbed by the restless hand of the rider without the use of driving aids.

The harmony of the aids and, therefore, throughness can only be assured by the rider's seat. Whether the rider sits erect or leans slightly forward, is of secondary importance. The most important aspect is that the rider sits into the movement of the horse. This means that the rider's legs feel and encourage the movement of the hindquarters, that the seat of the rider is parallel to the direction of the fibers of the long back muscle and moves light and forward in the saddle against the withers, and that the rider's upper body and hand lets the movement that has been transferred forward – forward thrust – out with the reins in a straight line to the horse's mouth. In racing, one can especially clearly observe how the rider lets the movement of the canter stride out forward in the final sprint to the finish. If one looks only at the rider's hands, it looks as if they push the horse forward in every stride with rigid reins. This following of the movement is not so obvious in the other gaits, but the basic principle of letting the thrust of the hindquarters out in the direction of the horse's mouth remains the same. Therefore, the half-halt may not be given at the moment when the hind leg pushes off from the ground because then two forces, two movements, would work against each other; however, the forward movement would always remain the stronger one and the rider would merely pull as hard as they could on the reins. In contrast, the horse is not able to use any force against the half-halt in the supporting phase and, therefore, it may be given only in this moment. Yet, this cannot be achieved by any rhythmic hand or arm movements, rather, this half-halt in the supporting flexion phase of the movement can only emerge from an elastically (positively) tensed rider's back as a result of a supple seat. During the half-halt, the rider should "sit against the bit." The half-halt thus acts in the moment the rider sits most deeply in the saddle in the supporting flexion phase and, if the rider sits into the movement of the horse, the rider's hand and the back give a little again as the horse pushes off. If the horse is on the driving aids and the rider sits into the movement, the even rein contact will maintain the speed, the accentuated following of the forward movement and, connected to it, giving with the hand in the pushing off phase will increase the speed by extending the steps or canter strides, and sitting lightly against the reins will shorten the steps or strides. Horses which are ridden in such a sensitive manner are "on the seat," which means they react only to the seat aids; in this case, rein contact only achieves the carriage.

It hardly needs to be stressed that only the perfect seat aspired to in the doctrines of riding makes this fine influence possible. In this seat, the rider's body is one unit which sits in the middle of the "bow" that is the horse. The driving leg aid bends (spans) the bow behind the saddle at will. The rein aid controls the elasticity generated at the back by means of the bow in front of the saddle; it restrains it or lets it out completely. The rider's back sits like a spring between the hand and the leg, connects, balances, and allows a seamless transition from one aid to another like a clutch. Riders' mistakes in seat and posture, especially the uncoordinated use of the arms with lowered hands and sitting back against the movement, disturb the unity in giving the aids and, thus, the harmony of the movement.

Although, at first glance, the jumping or racing seat appear to have little in common with the dressage seat, the basic effect of the seat and weight aids is the same. The balancing and elastic power of the rider's back is transferred by the closed knees of the rider to the horse in the same forward direction as the seat aid; and during energetic forward riding, for example just before a fence, we often see that the rider cannot do without sitting deeply in the saddle. This also results in a stronger flexion in the haunches, leading to elevation and increased take-off power (elasticity); the rider says that "the horse shortens itself."

We have to briefly mention the "sustaining or retaining rein aid," the combination of a sustaining rein aid and a stronger use of the driving leg aid in the same moment. One often sees that riders place their hands on the crest and drive their horse against the rein; they ride it forward until, in the process, it becomes light in the hand. These riders lack the strength to sit against the rein by using their back or the understanding of how the aids interact. The horse should not become light in the hand but on the rider's seat; the neck muscles should stretch in a supple manner, and the bars of the horse's mouth should maintain contact with the bit. The reins connect the horse's mouth through the hand with the elastically tensed back of the rider, whereby this line is the string for the stretched bow of the head and neck. The feeling of the elastic connection or so-called “elastic band” between the horse’s mouth and the rider’s hand can only be realized with an elastically tensed back. This elastic connection in the front can only be maintained and result in throughness if the driving leg makes the supporting hind leg flex. The rider’s back is the point where the movement is transferred onwards but where it can also get stuck. Driving the horse forward while using a sustaining rein aid is only good if the rider uses their seat aids to support the rein aid.

To reconcile contact, thoroughness, and carriage according to the horse’s level of training and to adjust the power of the hindquarters so that the movement remains natural and ground-covering, is, ultimately, a matter of the rider’s feel. The rider must acquire this feel through experience. Knowing the effect of the aids on the movement mechanics in the horse’s body will make this task easier.

8

Self-Carriage

a) Self-Carriage and Elevation

When the amateur says "the horse carries itself," they mean that it carries its neck in a raised position, in an upward convex arch, and it bends its head in the throat latch. From the sections entitled "How does the horse cope with the rider's weight?" and "The regulating aids" we know that this position is not a bend in the neck, independent of the body, but that it is rather determined by the shape and movements of the back, by the movements of the forehand, and the flexion in the hindquarters. Self-Carriage has a function; it is essential to carry the weight of the rider and for "throughness." Therefore, it must be relative to the horse's conformation, the level of its training, and the intended use of the horse.

The jumping and eventing horse needs its neck to balance the weight of its body over its forehand; therefore, the rein contact must allow a great deal of freedom in the neck. In extremely difficult terrain, it is more advisable for inexperienced riders to completely release the rein contact and let the horse cope on its own rather than obstruct it with incorrect rein aids, making it impossible for the horse to stretch its neck naturally.

Elevation (raise of the forehand) is required of the riding school horse. Equestrian literature refers to relative and active elevation. In simple terms this means: the relative raise of the forehand corresponds to the level of the horse's training; it is limited in young horse in its second year of training (Figure 17) and increases in relation to the flexion of the haunches (Figure 18). In principle, the function of the stretched muscles of the upper neck as described in Chapter 2 remains intact in relative elevation; the back swings and such horses allow the rider to sit comfortably. There is no shortening of the neck; the lower line of the neck remains concave, in maximum elevation at least straight; the horse's forehead is on or just in front of the vertical (Figure 18). Active raise of the forehand is an independent action of the muscles of the neck, actively lifting of the head with the upper neck muscles.

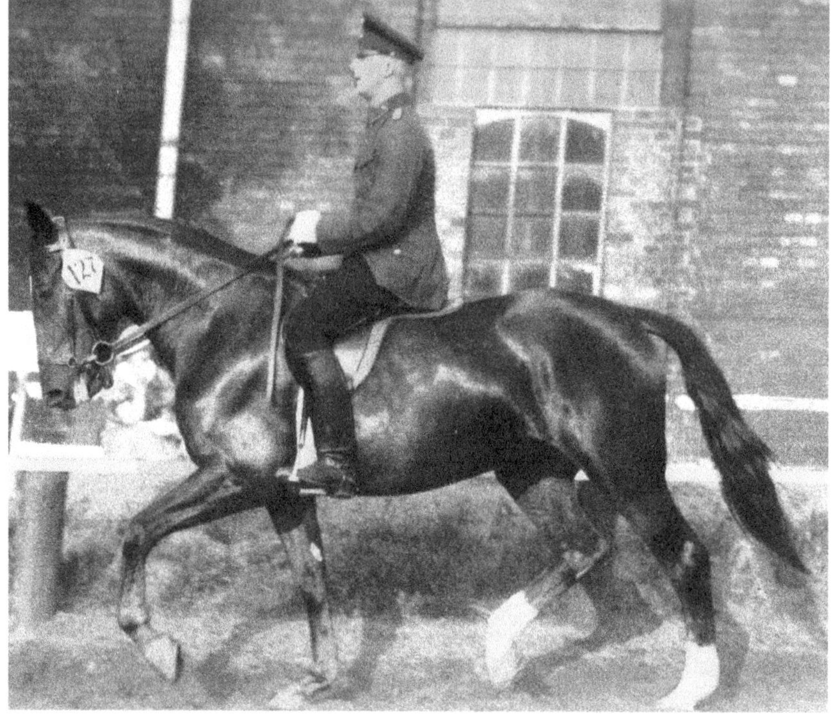

Figure 17: Posture of a horse in its second year of training without elevation

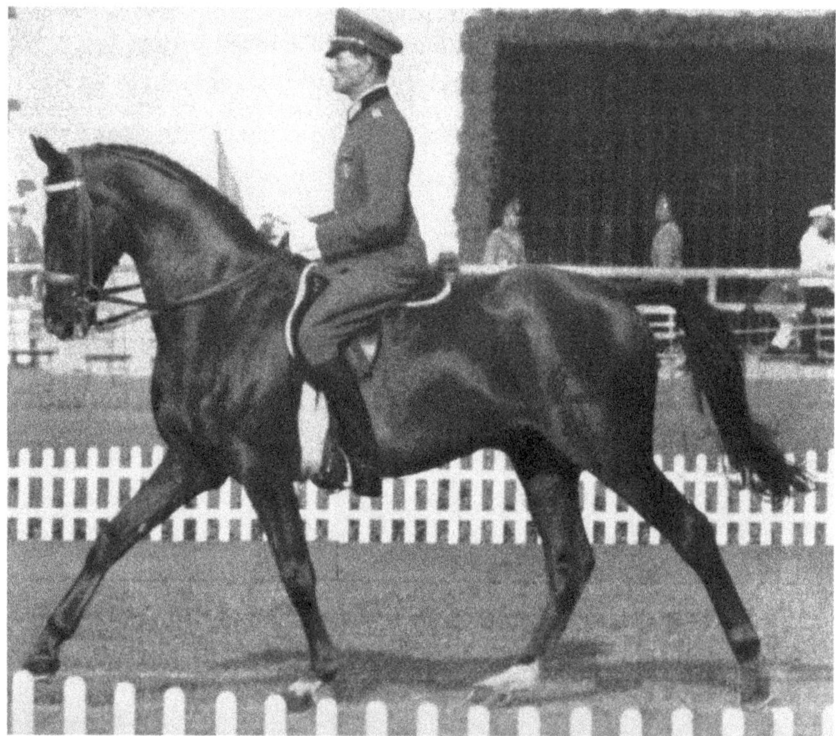

Figure 18: Highest possible elevation (relative raise of the forehand)

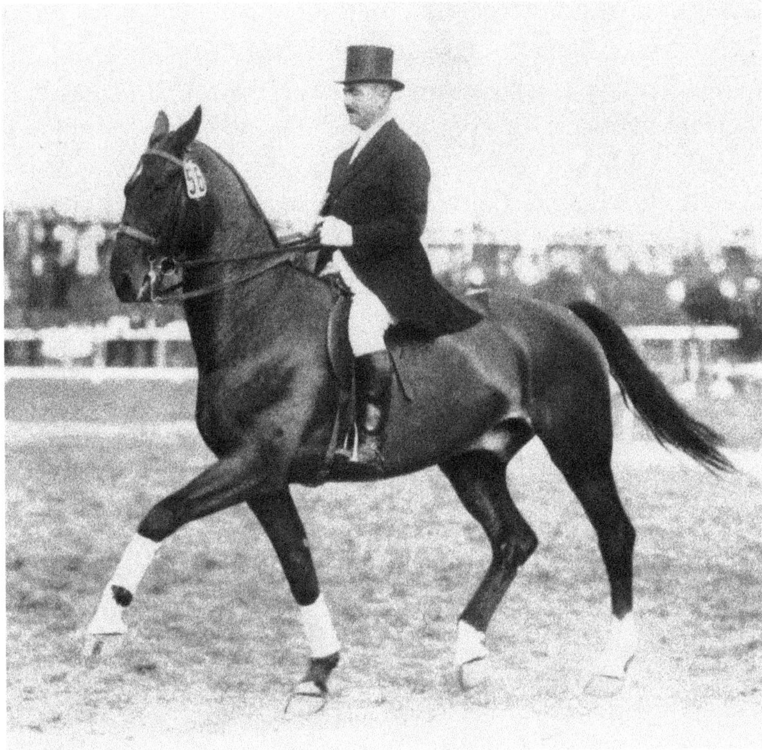

Figure 19: "Active" elevation (raise of the forehand)

The whole neck is more or less compressed, becomes shorter and takes the shape of an S; the cervical spine stands almost vertically and the lower outline of the neck forms a convex bulge (Figure 19). This unnatural posture cannot be compensated for by the flexion in the throat latch, so the forehead remains considerably in front of the vertical. The functional link between the upper neck muscles and the back is broken in this position; in trot the rider is jolted high out of the saddle. It requires no further explanation as to why only the relative raise of the forehand is desirable. To what extent the neck muscles are also actively involved in the relative raise of the forehand is explained in section c) which follows.

b) Nodding Movements

The supple horse which is walking forward freely makes a slight nodding movement with the neck at every step, i.e., it lifts the neck a little as it steps forward with a foreleg and lowers its neck again as it sets the foot down, to lift it again as the other foreleg steps forward etc. A horse which desperately tenses its neck muscles stiffens the neck and does not make these movements. In such horses, the movement in walk, trot, and canter is less ground-covering. These movements originate from the upper connection of the neck with the torso and shoulder on the one hand, and from the lower connection with the forelimbs on the other hand. The three large muscles of the upper neck, in addition to their attachment on the spine, have their origin in the withers-shoulder sheet, which moves together with the back and shoulder. As the foreleg is swung forward, this point of origin is moved backward with the upper part of the shoulder-blade, thus exerting a pull on the evenly stretched upper neck muscle and the neck is raised. The lower connection between the neck and foreleg is established by means of the head-neck-arm muscle (Figure 4, i, see Page 33). At its points of origin in the head and neck, this muscle joins the large spleen-shaped upper neck muscle (Figure 4, e); from here it extends along the cervical spine to the shoulder joint and the front surface of the humerus. By lifting the neck, the point of action of the head-neck-arm muscle is transferred forward-upward, the muscle is stretched prior to contraction, increasing its lifting height and the stride of the foreleg becomes more ground-covering.

In the young horse, the "nodding movements" are essential for unimpeded muscular activity. If the rider impedes the horse's nodding movements, the quality of its movement is inevitably lost. Over the course of consistent training, the muscles mentioned above increase in size and strength through training growth and are able to carry out the same job by actively contracting without obvious movement of the neck. In correctly ridden and trained horses, this nodding movement becomes also more apparent if they are extremely tired. The rider then has the opposite feeling, as if the foreleg which is set down and standing back is pulling the head, lowered from fatigue, down from the head-neck-arm muscle. These horses hardly lift their forelegs and tend to stumble.

For any trainer, preserving a free natural movement is the criterion for fixing and later raising the neck. In this respect, they pay particular attention to the walk on the bit. The walk can only be ground-covering if the neck muscles are supple and well-developed.

c) How the Neck is Suspended on the Withers and the Flexion in the Throat Latch

If we talk about stretching and bending of the neck and, consequently, about extensors and flexors, physiologically speaking, this correctly applies to the general free movements of the neck; these terms, however, tell us nothing about the function of this group of muscles in the riding horse. Without doubt, a riding horse should carry its neck in a rounded position. But if the flexor muscles which lie below the cervical spine played a significant role in this process, these would have to increase in size through exercise over the course of training; the lower (ventral) part of the neck would have to become larger. The opposite is the case: the flexor muscles decrease in size, the neck becomes thinner below the jugular vein.

The extensor muscles, or rather upper neck muscles, are, by comparison, naturally many times larger and experience a considerable growth in size during training. Therefore, even not very sensitive riders should have no doubt that the upper neck muscles do all the work: they carry the head and neck. Three muscles, reinforced with tendons, serve this purpose, two of which carry the neck and one the head. The muscles which carry the neck (the long neck muscle and the muscle of the withers, Figures 4, c and d, see Page 33) originate on the withers-shoulder sheet and the thoracic vertebrae and extend to the 7th to 4th cervical vertebra. In the naturally S-shaped neck, these muscles attach in a lower arch, with a concave shape upwards. If the horse stretches or lowers its neck, the lower part of the cervical spine hangs on these muscles. As these muscles become stronger during the course of training, their purely static or holding function increasingly becomes an actively carrying one. The muscles are then in a state of increased tension. They thus lift the 7th to 4th cervical vertebra to the withers, whereby the previously concave arch is stretched, the neck loses its S-shape and an attractive, regular upward convex arch develops. The neck becomes longer as a consequence.

The head is carried by the strong supporting muscle of the head (Figure 4, a). This has a broad origin on the withers-shoulder sheet and on the thoracic and cervical vertebrae and extends with a strong tendon to the occipital bone, becoming narrower in its course. Its base on the cervical spine is mobile, therefore, its state of tension depends on the muscles described before, the carrying muscles of the neck. The supporting muscle of the head has a purely static function in the posture of the riding horse, it is the suspensory apparatus of the head; therefore, it works in a state of passive extension and not in a state of active contraction. If the horse simply lets its head drop without actively bending, this muscle hangs on the extended muscle and the nuchal ligament; the upper neck becomes as long as it possibly, inevitably followed by the relaxed flexion in the throat latch. Hence, the supporting muscle of the head controls the posture of the head and the muscles which carry the head determine to what extent the neck is raised.

From what has been mentioned before, it is already clear that the flexor muscles of the neck on the lower part of the cervical spine play a subsidiary role. The horse should neither actively bend the neck as a whole nor the Atlanto-occipital joint[4]. If it did so, it would become tight in the neck and "heavy in the hand" in the first case, and, in the second, evade the bit by actively flexing in the throat latch and come behind the bit. The flexor muscles are certainly involved in lowering and rounding the neck, but never have to overcome any significant resistance, because the antagonists, the upper neck muscles, are themselves in a state of extension. The rein can be seen to assume the function of the flexor muscles. Due to this lack of

[4] The atlanto-occipital articulations function as bilaterally symmetrical ellipsoid synovial joints between C0 and C1. - *Physiopedia*. - Editor's note.

activity, we can observe a decrease in the size of these muscles and the whole section of the neck below the cervical spine becomes slimmer in correctly ridden horses.

d) Freedom of Movement in the Neck and its Importance for the Movement of the Forehand

The spleen-shaped muscle (Figure 4, e, see Page 33) is the large muscle of movement of the upper neck. Its origin is on the spinous processes of the withers and the withers-shoulder sheet, and it is also connected by an equally broad base to the occipital bone and to the 3rd to 5th cervical vertebra. The strong body of the muscle is completely fleshy; from which it can be concluded that it cannot have any static function.

The point where the spleen-shaped muscle attaches to the head and neck is, in essence, the origin of the head-neck-arm muscle (Figure 4, i), the muscle which swings the front leg forward; from here it extends to the front part of the humerus. The same area of origin determines a considerable degree of interdependence of both muscles. By lifting the neck, the spleen-shaped muscle transfers the point of action of the head-neck-arm muscle forward-upward; it thereby stretches this muscle and gives the foreleg a greater range of movement. However, a precondition for lifting the head correctly is that its position has been established as described in section c). If this is not the case, a contraction of the spleen-shaped muscle results in the unpleasant shaking of the horse's head, whereby the rider literally sees the nuchal ligament beneath the crest in serpentine loops before him. Constantly carrying the head by the spleen-shaped muscle results in an ewe neck, which in itself entails a shortening of the neck as well as results in the horse hollowing its back (letting it sag).

The interconnection of both these muscles, therefore, makes the movement of the forehand depend on the position of the neck (see Appendix, the brachiocephalic muscle). When the horse lands after a jump or even stumbles, the foreleg can only be brought far forward if there is total freedom of movement in the neck. These muscles working together on a neck which has been formed by correct training is extremely important for maintaining balance and, therefore, also for the horse to be sure-footed across country. These movements of the neck can also be seen in canter to a lesser extent; however, they can be even more distinctly felt by the rider.

e) Natural Crookedness, Straightening, Lateral Bend of the Longitudinal Axis of the Horse and Flexion

"Ride your horse forward and straighten it" is one of the basic requirements of the principles of riding. It is indeed rare that a horse naturally maintains straightness. One therefore talks about the "innate" crookedness, which manifests itself in the horse being slightly bent to one side through its entire body. People believe this to be the result of the position of the foal in the womb, but there is no proof of this.

This theory is contradicted by the fact that animals which give birth to multiple young are also crooked. This is especially obvious in the dog. It is also well-known that the two halves of the human body are very differently developed (right-handedness, varying step lengths when blindfolded).

One certainly does not err, if this lack of control over one's body and limbs is quite correctly attributed to the fact that all movements for specific purposes are always carried out identically and consequently become a habit. The same train of thought always initiates the same movement. During growth, the body unconsciously conforms to the few primitive movements and develops more or less one-sidedly. But later, when free will in the case of human beings or external force in the case of animals influence the movements of the body or limbs, these movements can become versatile and develop agility according to need. We shall probably never be able to explain why in most living beings the right half of the body is naturally more skilled than the left. It is, however, certain that both halves can achieve the same dexterity through exercise.

To overcome natural crookedness and, thus, straighten the horse is one of the most difficult hurdles in the training of a horse. The great majority of horses is bent to the right and they find it difficult to make the left side of the body hollow in the turn to the left. Therefore, horses turn quite happily to the right and yield willingly to the aid of right rein. However, they stiffen in a left-hand turn, remain bent to the right with the entire body, and resist the rein. In doing so, the hindquarters do not follow the track of the forehand but push into the turn, while the head and neck try to remain counter-flexed. On the circle, the horse pushes sideways against the inside leg toward the center of the circle.

Such a horse makes riders sit crookedly; it makes them sit deeper on the right side than the left. The experienced rider places more weight in the left stirrup and remains sitting straight, beginners are easily misled into lengthening the left stirrup by one or two holes because it seems to them to be too short. By lengthening the stirrup, they are thus able to sit again in the center of the horse's back, but to compensate for the differing stirrup lengths, the beginner rider has to collapse in the right hip and gets used to sitting crookedly. Hence, when a trainer notices a student's collapsed hip from behind, the trainer knows that the horse is not straightened. Any corrective measure must serve to straighten the horse, only then will the student be able to sit straight on the horse.

How does one straighten the horse? The precondition is that the horse willingly obeys the driving aids in a straight line, goes actively forward, and that the rein contact is reasonably established. Only then can one start to ask the horse to bend. Working on the circle with unilateral aids is crucial here. As the inside rein flexes the horse on the circle, the rider's inside leg uses strong pressure to make the horse, which tends to push toward the centre of the circle, hollow on the inside and to keep it on the circle line. The rider later applies the leg aid even more and pushes the horse toward the outside (increasing the size of the circle!), while maintaining the bend, so that the inside hind leg is forced to step over the outside hind leg. The outside rein should not be used at all at the beginning of this exercise. The diagonal aids (inside leg – outside rein) are much more difficult for the horse to understand.

Once the horse willingly obeys the one-sided sideways driving aids on the circle, these can be practiced alternately on a straight line. Very gradually, the contact will transfer from the inside to the outside rein, which is when the horse will learn the diagonal aids. A horse, which the rider has framed between their legs in a way that it allows itself to be bent equally to both sides and whose head and neck flexion follows the bend along the longitudinal axis of the body, is also straight. The hindquarters follow the track of the forehand. **Straightening is ultimately nothing other than a symmetrical development of both halves of the body with regard to strength and agility.**

Riding "in flexion" can also be misunderstood and overdone. The bend of the longitudinal axis of the horse is set by the inside leg and not by the rein. If the rider flexes their horse to the left, they see that the crest flips over to the left, to the inside, because this is the shorter side. This is the maximum degree of sideways bend when riding in flexion on a straight line. The bend in the neck must not be greater than the bend in the horse's entire body. If the rider seeks a stronger sideways flexion, they only pull the neck to the left, thus restricting the forward stride of the near foreleg; the horse takes irregular steps and may get into the habit of so-called bridle lameness.

Riding with the horse bent along its longitudinal axis as well as leg-yielding are exercises which extend beyond just straightening the horse by making use of the shortening of the steps and strides of the foreleg in horses that try to escape the driving aids by rushing forward. The experienced rider is able to apply driving aids in these movements, increases the activity of the hind leg, and allows the steps of the forehand to come through freely and evenly with soft use of the reins. The unskilled rider, who simply flexes the horse forcibly with the reins and does not ride forward at all or too little, may take away the horse's desire to go forward and destroy its movement for ever.

9

To What Extent Can the Evaluation of Muscular Development Determine the Course of Training of the Riding Horse?

There are experienced riders and equine experts who, with unerring precision, can pick out the horses which have been correctly ridden from a group of horses shown in hand. Primarily, it is the general conformation that is the determining factor for them. In addition, they evaluate the definition of the most important muscular groups characteristic for the riding horse. These experts are also able, without seeing a horse under saddle, to specify what difficulties it will probably present when ridden, because they see which muscle groups are still undeveloped. They draw conclusions as to which corrective or training exercises will be required to strengthen the affected muscle groups and to eliminate the problems. It is advisable for every young rider to train their eye in this respect. Every time riders are about to get onto an unfamiliar horse, they should take a careful look and consider what kind of ride to expect. On the other hand, riders must look at the state of muscular development of all the horses of their string, whose strengths and weaknesses the rider knows well. It is the only way to gather the experience which is needed to evaluate the **riding** horse. The rider will learn to differentiate between major conformation faults and so-called "excusable faults" which can be compensated by developing general muscle strength and individual muscle groups. The rider will also abandon to work all horses according to the same program. Rather, the rider will, more appropriately, establish a training program and individual exercises tailor-made for each horse. No objections should be made because this may be too complex or even time-consuming. The opposite is true. By working horses individually, they will progress much more quickly, so that it is easy to later put together a group of well-schooled horses. The basic principle for a successful education program is to establish a healthy balance of training and dressage. The trainer must see which muscle groups are poorly defined and need to be developed. The trainer must be able to judge whether the problems which arise lie with the horse or the rider. If they are to be found in the horse, the trainer should be able to suggest the right corrective measures or exercises which will compensate for these problems, with the goal to primarily develop the weak muscle groups. Initially, exercises must be selected which are most natural and easiest for the horse. For example: strength in the hindquarters can be developed by means of numerous dressage exercises: through turns on the haunches, rein back followed immediately by trot, shoulder-in, gymnastic work in hand etc.; in essence through exercises to make the haunches flex. If the rider does not have the necessary sensitivity for this, it can be achieved through repeated canter transitions, long steady canters, and climbing. Average riders will thus achieve their goal much sooner and more efficiently and, later, be in a position to ask for dressage exercises from the strengthened hindquarters which previously would have resulted in resistance on the part of the horse.

To facilitate evaluation of muscular development, there follows a summary of the characteristics of the badly and well-developed muscles with short notes on appropriate compensation exercises. This is an excerpt from all the chapters, the common thread which runs through this book.

The Neck

Poor musculature: prominent cervical spine with the head-neck-arm muscle located on its side; clearly defined flexor muscles of the head and neck; sunken lateral muscles of the upper neck; large triangular indentation between the cervical spine, the base of the neck, and the crest. Seen from the rider's perspective above, the neck is widest at the level of the cervical spine and becomes too narrow toward the crest.

Good musculature: The muscles of the upper neck are so well-defined that the cervical spine does not protrude above them. The triangle described before is filled out by the training growth of the upper neck muscles and the connecting muscles to the shoulder. The latter are always especially well-developed in correctly ridden horses. This is visible in a clearly defined muscle bulge above the cervical spine and in front of the base of the neck, seemingly emerging from the front edge of shoulder. The flexor muscles in front of the cervical spine are poorly developed, the neck and throat latch are "dry" (exposed), and the jugular vein is very clearly visible. Seen from above, the neck above the cervical spine is widest in the area of the upper neck muscles.

Guidelines for developing the neck muscles: riding forward with a stretched neck in a light contact. Fundamentally, the muscles of the upper neck are working correctly when the horse goes actively forward, stretches its neck, relaxes, and employs its back, allowing the rider to sit. The neck then takes shapes of its own accord. Directly working the neck muscles in any way is wrong from the point of view of the rider; this work depends entirely on a supple back and a free natural movement.

The back

Poor musculature: The long muscle of the back is flat or even sunken in, the spine is very prominent not only in the saddle area but also in the region of the loins.

Good musculature: The long back muscle entirely fills the region of the loins and reaches the level of the spine. In movement, one can observe the muscle working alternately on both sides; the side which is arching up can become so high that, seen from the side, the muscle rises above the level of the spine.

Guidelines for developing the back muscles: suppleness of the back; free, rhythmic movement; repeated canter transitions from trot and long periods of canter; changes of speed; cavaletti; uneven terrain and climbing inclines.

The Hindquarters

Poor musculature:
Seen from the side: flattened croup; the muscle which supports the patella is caved in; the long muscles of the *ischium* are not prominently visible beneath the skin; the line of the buttock is straight. In general, the thigh of an unfit horse is flat; the contours of the bulging muscles are missing.
Seen from behind: flat croup; flat thighs; a big cleft between the thighs; poor, flat muscles on the side of the lower thigh (calf muscle).

Good musculature: round, convex croup; the muscles of the thighs bulge visibly and the grooves between the muscles stand out beneath the skin; the line of the buttocks is convex, the space between the thighs is small (inner long muscles of the *ischium*); seen from behind, the calf muscle bulges more visibly to the outside.

Guidelines for developing the muscles of the hindquarters: all collecting exercises described in the Principles of Riding, also long canters, frequent transitions to canter, riding in uneven terrain and climbing uphill (Figures 6 and 7, Pages 42/43). The more this natural way of moving is made use of, the less resistance the average rider will encounter.

The Forehand

Poor musculature: The outlines of the shoulder blade stand out clearly during movement; the scapular spine is clearly visible and palpable. There is a deep indentation in front of the entire length of the shoulder blade if the connecting muscles to the neck are poorly developed. The muscles in the angle of the shoulder joint between the shoulder blade and upper arm up to the point of the elbow (the extensor of the elbow, broad back muscle) are flat; the entire circumference of the forearm is small.

Good musculature: The contours of the shoulder blade are covered by muscles; the scapular spine is embedded in the shoulder muscles which extend above it. The front connecting muscles (suspensory muscles of the ribs, neck section of the serrated muscle, thorax-shoulder muscle, head-neck-arm muscle) are so well-defined, that the neck appears to be broadly set on the shoulders. The elbow extensors bulge out strongly between the shoulder blade and the elbow. The broad back muscle fills the dent between the shoulder and outward curve of the ribs and allows for the saddle to lie well on the horse. The front muscles on the forearm should protrude bulbously, the ones at the rear should reach the vertical line from the point of the elbow downward and not be constricted below the elbow. These forearm muscles can be considered as the benchmark of judging the stability of the forehand. Their development must be especially carefully monitored and should be the determining factor for increasing the demands when jumping young horses. Although there is no proof that the durability of tendons depends on the strength of the forearm muscles, the well-trained forearm certainly lets us conclude that the tendons have also become stronger during the course of this training. Judging the forehand as a whole is the most difficult thing to do, but that of the forearm muscles alone is very easy and the conclusions are reliable. In the case of an untrained eye, measurements taken at extended intervals with a tape measure are helpful. In a 5-year-old horse with poor muscles of the forearm, we have measured an increase of 5cm in circumference over the course of one year.

Guidelines for developing the muscles of the forehand: Our dressage riders are living proof that movement with impulsion strengthens the muscles of the forearm as part of general fitness. The average rider, unfortunately, does not have the same success. Most periods of forced rest for their horses are injuries to the forehand as a result of excessive strain. Therefore, one must also systematically exercise the forehand and not just expect it to hold up if a horse is 6 years old before it is taken hunting or possibly show-jumping. This is even more so, if the conformation of the forelegs or musculature leaves something to be desired. Good musculature can compensate for some conformation defects (e.g. sloping pastern). Strengthening the forehand is most easily achieved by working for longer periods, long hacks, long, steady canters, climbing, riding in uneven terrain, and many very easy jumps. Calm and fluent movement in all gaits and especially when riding over fences is the main prerequisite to avoid bruises of the forehand as only these can result in injuries, as well as exhaustion in canter, which can certainly be avoided during training.

The Abdomen

It is difficult to describe musculature as good or poor in this area. A "compact" horse should have a belly, i.e. the flanks should be round and well-filled out. We want neither an excessively bulging, drooping belly with a "sunken" *Paralumbar fossa* between the last rib and the coxal tuberosity (point of the hip), nor do we want a constricted belly with a wasp waist. We can, however, be forced to make do with horses with such faults. The large or so-called hay belly is the lesser of two evils in young horses. Frequently, it is simply a sign of still being foal-like, the animal is not yet fully mature. As general fitness improves, and the abdominal muscles in particular strengthen, the hay belly disappears with consistent training. On no account should one attempt to hasten this process by reducing the quantity of roughage.

It is not always easy to evaluate the constricted abdomen. Usually, these horses have been underfed when they were young, or at least been fed too little roughage. The intestinal tract has not developed sufficiently, the abdominal cavity has remained correspondingly small. Everything possible must be done for these horses to get them used to consuming larger quantities of roughage. It is possible to make up for some of the damage until the 6th year of a horse's life. If young horses with very constricted abdomens are also badly muscled, they are ill or receiving inadequate amounts of feed, they must be fed and treated, but not ridden.

This short summary does not mean that the separate chapters should not be read; only reading each section in depth will enable the reader to appreciate the full picture. At the end of this section, we must repeat, just like in the introduction, that one can never completely judge a horse simply by looking at it. The horse's innate constitution plays a most important role. One can certainly develop each individual horse on the basis of personal observations; but one cannot compare the ability to perform and robustness of different animals with each other simply on the grounds of variations in muscular development. There is no substitute for testing performance.

10

Suppleness

It has been repeatedly mentioned in the previous sections that muscles should be "supple". This term still has to be explained. A great deal has already been written about it, but all the theoretical studies cannot be of any help to a rider who has never sat on a perfectly supple horse. A feeling for suppleness can only develop in the saddle. The rhythmic movement with impulsion, the swinging back, the stretching of the neck, and the rein contact are aspects which always result from suppleness; however, some of these can also be observed in horses which quite obviously are not supple. For example, we see horses winning advanced dressage classes, obeying the rider's most subtle aids, and yet, the rider's seat pounds the saddle audibly and visibly in medium trot. Such a back is certainly not supple; the horse's presentation is very tense; the harmony is lacking. If one said "harmony of movement" instead of suppleness and "involuntary tension" instead of the horse working with a tight and tense back, we would have two expressions which every amateur understands because sport trainers use them every day on the sports field, during gymnastics, and exercise programs. If one watches people doing gymnastics, it is not difficult to notice enormous differences in the way they move. Everyone wants to accomplish the same movements; some people appear natural, graceful, harmonious while doing so, others clumsy, awkward, and grotesque. Some are supple (relaxed), the others tense. Involuntary tension is individual, not natural but more or less deeply rooted in a lack of suitable exercise of the body and reassured by a certain timidity of the mind, a lack of self-confidence. These physically tense people are often shy of raising their voices loudly; this is why experienced sports trainers often begin a so-called loosening exercise by making everybody shout loudly, because students lose their inner inhibitions by forcing themselves to shout. Getting rid of tension is the **ultimate aim** of physical exercise. What degree of suppleness can be attained, leaving circus acts aside, can be clearly seen in gymnastics. A dive roll over six men is a good average achievement at every military gymnastics display. Suppleness or tension is clearly obvious to the observant spectator in these complex exercises as well as all other movements such as running or walking. It is impossible to fully deploy strength in a state of tension. Suppleness is the precondition for perfect control over muscles, for involuntary suitable movements, for breathing freely; hence, in total, for individual optimum performance.

These observations with regard to humans have been made in such detail because it is inexplicable why the suppleness of the horse is often judged differently from that of the human being. The much quoted "horse in the pasture" can be supple or not. If one chases grazing horses about, one can observe that some of them canter away with beautiful, energetic, and harmonious movements, others with tense backs and short canter strides. From this, one cannot, however, draw any conclusions as to how these horses will become supple under a rider, since the temperament and sensitivity toward the rider play at least as great a role in a horse's readiness to supple as its physical predisposition. We like to assume that in young horses the unfamiliar sensation of the rider's weight generally results in a cramped muscular state, in rider's terms, "negative tension." The force which the horse experiences will be even greater if the rider interacts with it in an unnatural manner, and if the rider tries to impose their will on the horse in an awkward manner.

At the beginning of every training program, it is essential to familiarize the horse. It must be ingenious when in contact with humans, and must go forward naturally and rhythmically in hand, behind a lead horse, and potentially on the lunge. It must recognize the voice of its trainer and pay attention and obey commands such as walk, come, halt, come here, forward, no etc. on the lunge with pricked ears. Horses which still display tense gaits next to a lead horse and jump nervously and bolt on the lunge at each movement of the whip are not mentally supple. When a rider is mounting, these horses will also tense their back muscles; the force, stress, and nerves prevent them from being able to find a suitable way of holding themselves to lighten their load. If nothing has been neglected in the familiarization phase of training described before and the horse's movements and behavior are unconstrained, it will normally quietly permit the rider to get on its back for the first time. At most it may react by putting its head down, arching its back, kicking out strongly, or even bucking. The latter are absolutely appropriate supple defensive measures against the unknown weight on its back. Now the rider only needs to feel for the rhythm of the movement and make the horse go forward by means of light taps of the whip. The familiar voice and calming pats on the neck will soon make the horse understand that it is time to learn something new. Riders who know exactly how to handle young horses can immediately get on a horse without the preparatory stages. It is amazing what young horses which are used to people will accept if they are handled quietly but confidently. The better riders relieve the back and the more they follow the horse's natural movement, the less resistance they will encounter. Muscular suppleness can only follow if the horse approaches everything with an open mind. Every trainer should recognize the external signs of beginning suppleness. These are the rhythmic, free movement, the tail held straight and swinging evenly, snorting as a sign of unrestricted breathing, stretching the neck, often combined with swaying, balancing movements, the swinging back on

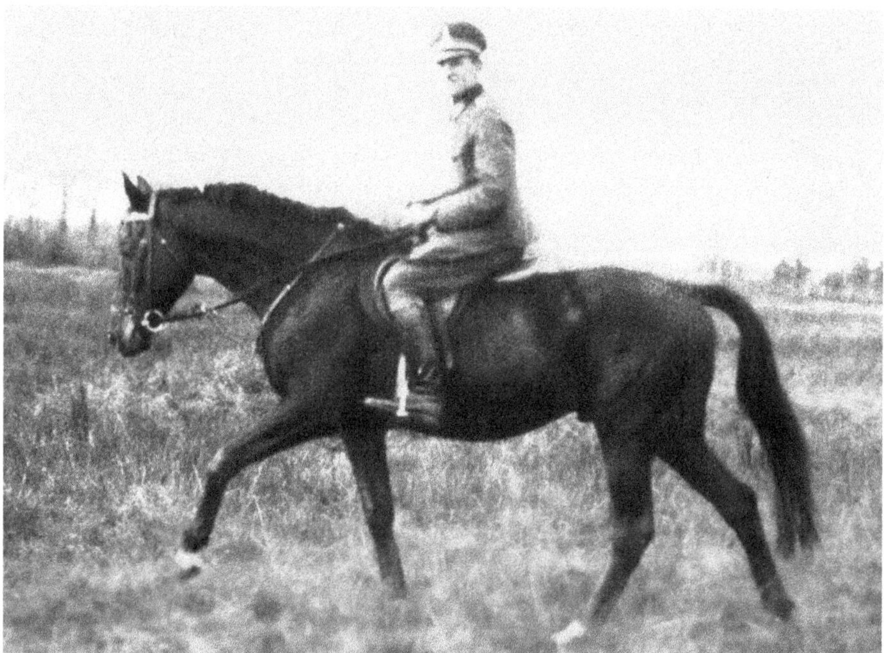

Figure 20: Suppleness (free walk on a long rein)

which the rider can sit comfortably, and the bucking of young horses in canter in the first two years of their training. The general impression of the horse is calm; the movements are fluid and harmonious (Figure 20). And to the opposite: the tense horse carries its neck stiffly, moves its ears nervously, the back is tense, so that the rider bounces strongly out of the saddle, the tail is pressed flat against the body or often held at a crooked angle, the movement is irregular, either too fast or restricted, dragging, the steps are of uneven length. But the worst consequences of tension are jogging and pacing.

Thus far, we have only talked about the young horse which should learn to become supple and use its muscles properly. This learning process can take a very long time, even years. In older horses under saddle, we differentiate between three types with respect to suppleness. The first are horses which have never learnt to "supple;" their upper neck and back muscles are visibly underdeveloped. The second are well-ridden and well-muscled horses but want to be ridden well with prominent aids to become supple and use their entire strength. Under an unskilled rider, these horses retain their incorrect tensions and go easy on themselves by avoiding free movement and flexing their haunches. The third are ideal riding horses which readily supple, balance themselves, and are willingly on the aids.

We are coming to the crucial point of our anatomical and functional observations in respect to suppleness. Only a horse which is supple uses its muscles properly, i.e., in the sense that it uses those muscles which are reinforced with tendinous fibers in a static function and the other muscles are available to perform forward movement,

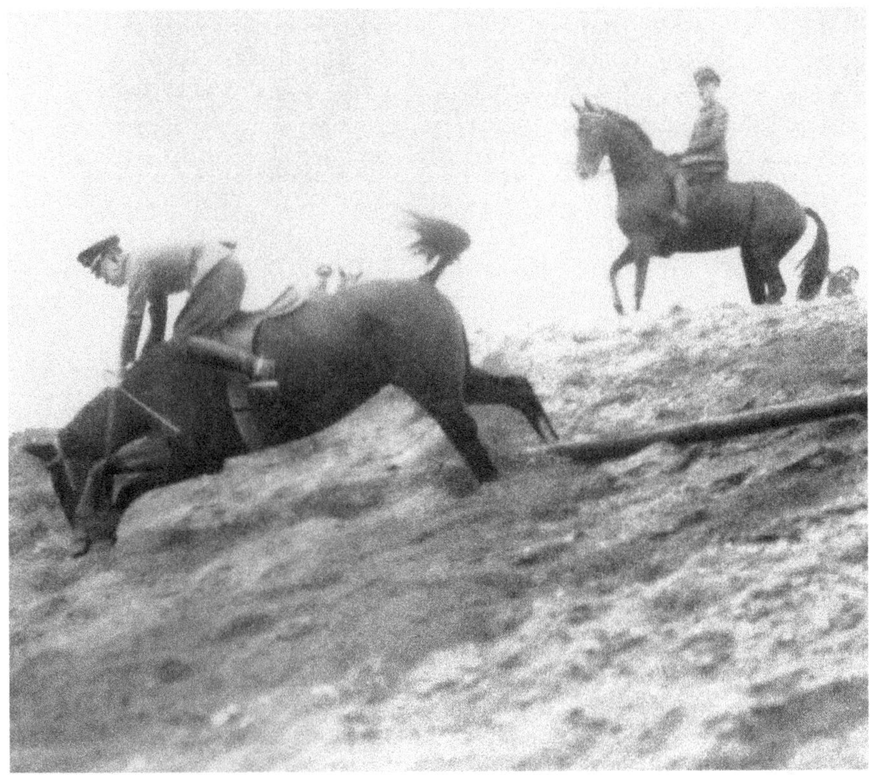

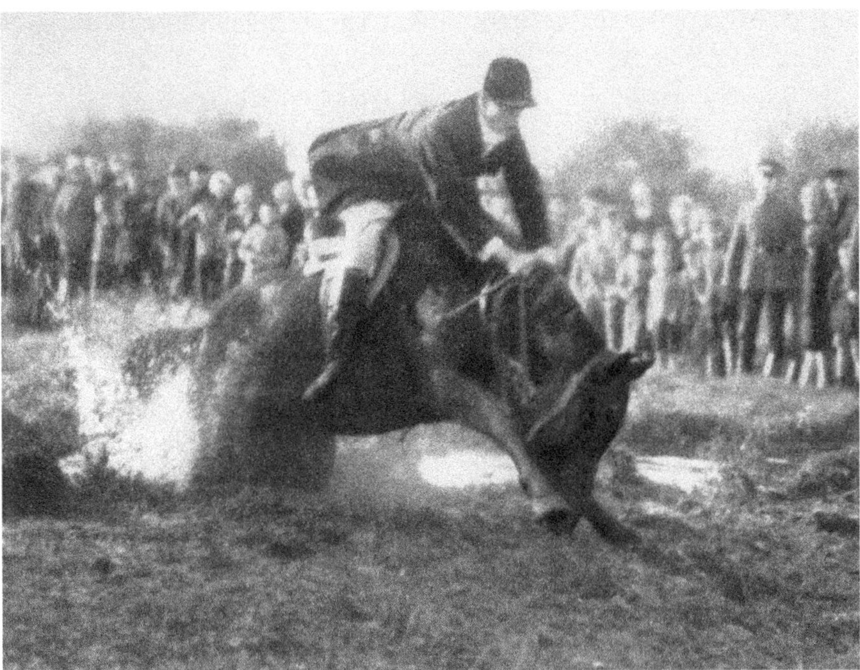

Figure 21 and 22: Stumbling. The horses continue to move forward, rest their noses on the ground, and put the left or right foreleg forward to stop themselves from falling. The riders remain skillfully in center of gravity of the horse.

jumping etc. If we differentiate between muscles which are used in a static manner and muscles of movement, then the correct use and orderly interaction of the static apparatuses allow the horse to carry itself under the rider with the least effort, while the unrestricted activity of the movement muscles permits the highest level of performance. Only muscles which are used functionally correct in this manner will become stronger through proper training and increase in size.

This is exactly why the suppleness of the horse is the foundation, the obvious starting point for a training program which has development of muscular strength as its goal. Every trainer knows that the rider's suppleness is the perquisite for the horse to be supple. To ride in difficult terrain across country, it is absolutely imperative that both horse and rider are supple. Only perfect control over all the muscles of the body and uninhibited concentration of all the senses on the terrain to be mastered make those appropriate involuntary movements possible which are often suddenly needed at confusing obstacles to avoid an impending fall or make it safe. How often do we see horses which are stumbling heavily, place their nose or forehead on the ground and bring a front leg forward to save themselves (Figures 21 and 22) while still moving forward, or horses, as they fall, bend their necks strongly and roll harmlessly over the crest and backs (Figure 23) as the rider, who is falling in just as supple a manner, takes a dive roll far in front of their falling horse. On the other hand, the tense horse and rider already brace themselves in anticipation of the fall as the horse loses control over its forelegs during the landing. And if the fall actually does occur, the horse lands on its chin with its head raised and, thereby, all too frequently, breaks its neck or back and the rider falls with hands outstretched onto their face or shoulder. For such tense riders and horses, riding across country will always remain an unsafe and dangerous experience no matter how often they practice. Suppleness is also of great importance in the work and performance of racehorses. In addition, experienced trainers see it as the surest way to prevent a horse from sustaining tendon injury (**Count Spreti**, in personal communication).

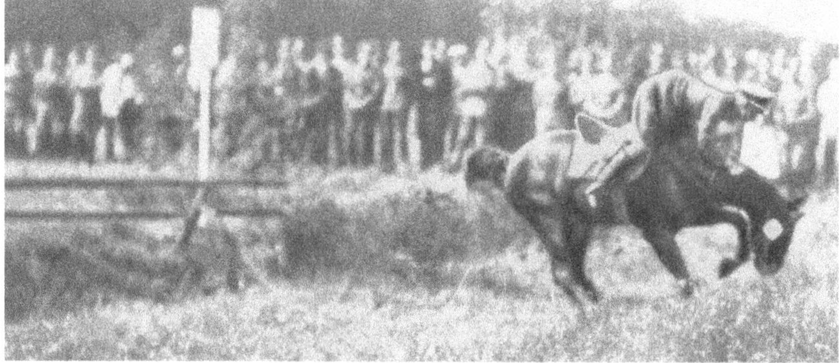

Figure 23: Stumbling. The horse braces itself with its hind legs against the fall. The rider is thrown forward as the horse stops. The fall is apparently inevitable, so the horse bends its neck down and to the left to roll in a supple manner over its right shoulder.

11

Balance

The old equestrian masters were of the opinion that a horse was naturally unbalanced because its body weight was distributed with approximately 5/9ths on the forehand and 4/9ths on the hindquarters. This led them to conclude that everything possible should be done in equitation to re-distribute the weight onto the hindquarters and relieve the forehand. Their aim was to place "equal weight" on all four feet; this was supposed to be achieved through collection – raising the neck, bringing the hind legs further under the body, and flexing the haunches. For centuries, a grotesque contortion of rider and horse resulted from unquestioning adherence to this doctrine and not even so long ago, there were riders who forced a military horse to land first with its hind legs after a fence, or at least land on all four feet simultaneously, with the rider actively assisting by leaning back and pulling sharply on the reins (Figures 9 and 10, see Page 49). The natural way of landing was considered to be the only harmful method because ostensibly too much weight was placed on the forehand. In spite of this theory, races and hunts were ridden at which the horses always landed on the forehand despite the best efforts of some of the riders to prevent the horses from doing this and, instead, putting their entire weight on their hindquarters. Nowadays, practical riding has long abandoned this contentious theory. Other expressions have been found for what the rider feels on a horse. The most accurate of these is the requirement that the rider "should sit into the movement." The rider leans forward in the direction of the forward movement when they want to go faster and sits more upright with their upper body when they want to bring the horse back.

In the supple horse, the outline of the rider's back always follows the movements of the horse's neck. The rider leans far forward when the horse stretches its neck forward and downward as it takes the jump (Figure 24). Conversely, the rider sits very upright as the horse moves in the raised head and neck self-carriage required in dressage (Figure 14, see Page 62). In spite of these changed views, nowadays, collection is still required of horses. The purpose of collection, however, is not to place more weight on the hindquarters but for the rider to have control of the horse's

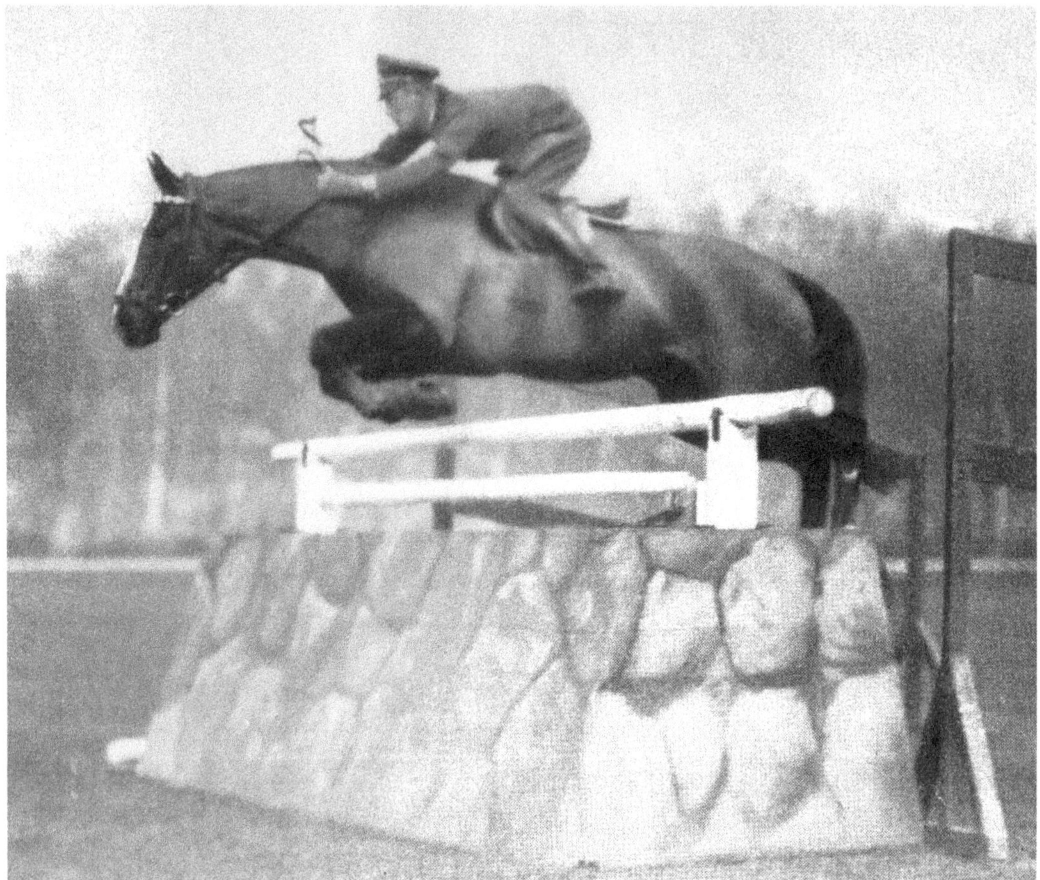

Figure 24: The rider sits into the movement. The curve of the rider's back follows the angle and extension of the neck of the horse.

hind legs (see Chapter 7). The dressage rider who works their horse in the highest degree of collection also sits up against the pommel of the saddle and uses the driving aids to activate the hindquarters to step forward and to flex the haunches. If the rider wanted to place more weight on the hindquarters, they would shift their weight toward the back. Flexing the haunches is intended to give the horse's movement more impulsion and give the rider a pleasant swinging feeling. Today, nobody thinks any more of taking the weight off the "fragile" forehand. The term "balance" in the sense of distributing the weight equally, is therefore incorrect. It is often said that a horse is naturally well-balanced. The Irish hunter is praised for this quality. In general, these are extremely well-muscled, short horses with rather long bodies with deep chests; in short, horses which carry considerably more weight on the forehand than on the hindquarters. Conversely, very tall horses with short bodies are seldom well-balanced. Experienced riders know exactly what is meant by these expressions. In the following section, we will attempt to explain this concept to the beginner.

The different functions of the muscles of the forehand and hindquarters have been described in the appropriate sections. The motor is positioned in the hindquarters, they propel the body mass forward; the forehand absorbs the weight and pushes it forward again. In a well-balanced horse, both these forces are equal. If the hindquarters are more strongly developed and more energetic, the horse "falls" on the forehand in movement and does not push off sufficiently afterwards. The movement is flat and dull. And vice versa, if the hindquarters are too weak compared to the forehand. In this case, thrust and elasticity are insufficient and the movement becomes short or sluggish. It is said that the horse is on the forehand and the hindquarters do not keep up. This makes it clear that the movement of the well-balanced horse is energetic, with impulsion, and confident. The horse makes the rider sit correctly, i.e., in its centre of gravity. The rider has the feeling that they have equal sources of power in front and behind the saddle, while in a badly balanced horse there is always an imbalance between these two forces. On a horse with a stronger forehand, the rider sits behind the movement in the horse's hollow back, if the hindquarters are stronger, the rider feels that more weight is tipping them forward. Being balanced, therefore, depends on even muscular development and is the result of training and exercise. It cannot be temporarily achieved by the re-distribution of the rider's weight; rather, the rider must always sit in the horse's centre of gravity, which is continuously changing in all the gaits.

12

Basic Principles of Training

It is often written in reports of the great sporting triumphs of top riders that only perfect harmony between horse and rider can produce such outstanding performances. This harmony should not be interpreted simply as a matter of technique but as harmony of movement; in addition, it is also a harmony of the mind, a spiritual bond between horse and rider. One may think what they like about the spiritual qualities of the horse – soul, ratio, or instinct – such arguments have only theoretical merit. For the observant rider, there is no question that all horses have a will of their own and that their level of comprehension varies enormously from one animal to another. Through training, the rider can achieve to forever turn the horse against them as a result of bad experiences; secondly, that the horse's will is broken and that it is taught passive sufferance and obedience; and thirdly, the ideal: the horse happily and trustingly uses all its strength, skill, and focus to carry out what the rider asks of it. The more intelligent the horse, the quicker it learns what is required of it. The only way this can be developed is through experience gained through a series of identical stimuli.

To present these stimuli in an identical manner over the course of a horse's education is the most important duty of the rider. This includes a feeling for total consistency, for clear aids, and, last but not least, equestrian skill in the saddle. Not all people have such a bond with their horses that they also think about keeping the horse happy. They do not know that riding the horse for long distances at speed contributes to its well-being; on the contrary, they find the rush of happy excitement which every horse experiences when it feels grass under its hooves quite uncomfortable. Dressage is an end in itself for these riders; they force the horse to hold itself in the prescribed carriage to have total control over it. They do not want to allow the horse to take attentive notice of its surroundings; they never leave the horse to itself so that it can move as nature intended. Only what is natural can be sensible and correct and only the horse which senses its surroundings consciously and understandingly, and which training is based on an unforced natural way of moving and of carrying itself can willingly produce optimum performance. The reader of this text can be in no doubt as to what this means.

The training of a riding horse comprises three areas: dressage, exercise, and obedience training. Each of these should be accorded equal importance.

It is not the purpose of this text to give overall training and lesson rules which can be read in the *Principles of Riding* and other equestrian literature. Here, we should compare the merits of the three areas mentioned above. We will try to clarify, in part, by means of examples, how these must complement each other if unnecessary problems and setbacks during training are to be avoided. Beyond the usual application of aids, the rider will discover a deep spiritual bond with their horse through these reflections; they will be able to differentiate between the horse "being able or willing" and then be in a position to either progress or implement corrective measures. The training of the military horse is long enough without getting bogged down in one-sidedness. The goal to train a capable, quiet, sensible, and, thus, reliable riding horse, can be achieved for any horse in two years.

At the beginning of training, the rider must gain the complete trust of their horse; only then can the horse learn to carry the rider, at first behind a lead horse, later to go forward on its own in a straight line, and to turn, following the sideways guiding rein. If the horse responds willingly, it will then not experience any unpleasant impressions. The next phase is the "education," the obedience training of the horse, developing its character. The horse must understand that the human being is its friend and not a nuisance. The relatively short time for which a horse leaves its stable should be a pleasure. A light hack is natural for all horses which have been used to being turned out when they were young. One should make use of this and hack out frequently, at first across country even in bad, hilly terrain or even terrain which has holes in the ground. The horse will thus be forced to pay attention to the footing and its surroundings and will accept a rider who sits lightly in the saddle and does not interfere, without finding the rider to be too much pressure. Deviations from natural movement such as hurrying, jogging, or restraint, which are always the result of some feeling of force, hardly ever happen. The rider should limit their influence to driving carefully with their legs and whip. Basically, the rider drives in all the gaits, while the regulating rein aids are used initially only for a downward transition into the next gait or to a halt. If necessary, these rein aids should be used very energetically. If this is successful, the rider must immediately give with the reins. In this way, the rider will avoid to pull tightly on the reins and problems in the throat latch will be avoided. Stopping often and letting the horse graze without dismounting before riding on brings the head and neck down and relaxes the masticatory muscles.

Once the horse goes forward willingly on the driving aids, rein contact should be offered to the horse. This must always be so light that the movement remains free and rhythmic. At this stage, correctly exercising the horse should be more important than specific dressage training. The rider has control of the horse to the extent that it can be ridden behind a lead horse at first and then, soon afterwards, anywhere alone, even through running water, over ditches, and appropriate obstacles. The following time should be used to encourage muscle growth by means of long hacks across country. This general strengthening of the horse makes the subsequent dressage work easier because the majority of problems which arise in the back and especially in the hindquarters as a result of insufficient strength will no longer occur.

Riding young horses on uneven terrain has another advantage: the tendons and especially the ligaments of the joints become strong. A person who for years has only been walking on city streets will most probably sprain their ankle if they have to walk across a plowed field. Exactly the same thing happens to horses which have been worked mostly on level arena footing when they were young and are later taken for their first canter across country. Occasional sprains of the tendons, ligaments, and muscles after the horse misses its footing do not cause any lasting injury in young horses; potential lameness is soon cured without leaving any trace. However, if the horse is lacking this sort of training in its younger years, serious tendon and joint injuries are all too easily sustained later on.

A word or two about developing the horse's character. The more impulsive a horse is, the more spirited it is, the more distinctly willful it is. But complete obedience is the basic requirement for a riding horse. If the horse is securely on the aids, this is equal to complete obedience in the eyes of a good rider. Obedience would then simply be a question of dressage training. It is, however, a well-known fact that poor riders are usually helpless on well-trained and spirited horses as these horses react to every mistake on the part of the rider with disobedience, resistance, or bolting.

The military horse does not always carry a good rider and, therefore, it should be taught to use a certain degree of independence from an early stage of training when it is hacked out. If one sometimes hears that people are of the opinion that a horse needs rein contact to go forward with balance and not stumble, then one must contradict this by saying that a training which results in such instability can only be wrong. The horse should go forward on a loose rein just as quietly, confidently, and energetically as with rein contact, and should remain on the driving aids without hurrying. It should notice obstacles in front of it in good time, appraise them attentively, and only then approach at a measured pace and jump. The horse should learn to deal with deep gullies and climbing sections primarily on its own without any rein contact.

Mistakes which defy the horse's nature can be seen much too often. In most cases, the rider does not differentiate between what a horse wants to do or is able to do. If young horses refuse an obstacle, it is wrong to punish them with a reinback.

This will only make their fear and stress even greater. If the horse is otherwise securely on the forward driving aids, it will jump at the second attempt without punishment after it has had a good look at the obstacle; otherwise, the lead horse must go first. If all fails, it is still better to give up the attempt for the time being until the horse is obedient again to the forward driving aids than to try to force it by means of a pointless, often rough struggle which only serves to cement a permanent fear of obstacles. Turning after an obstacle and jumping back over is a consistency error. The horse must know that it has to jump the ditch to continue straight. Competitively jumping a course in the arena may only be attempted once the horse can jump confidently on a straight line in open country.

A horse must be punished immediately, however, for obvious vices and for as long as it takes until the rider has the horse back on the aids. If, for example, a horse kicks out at the touch of the whip and stops, the rider must immediately respond with the whip again and release the rein until the horse goes or rushes forward; the rider must then praise the horse. This is being consistent. The horse which runs out in front of an obstacle should be pulled up very sharply facing the opposite side, i.e., to the obstacle, turned, and presented with the obstacle again in a direct line!

Habitual shying is a very unpleasant quality in a military horse. Young horses which go confidently under the rider seldom shy. They turn to face unfamiliar objects and look at them intensely. The rider should then remain totally passive but keep talking reassuringly to the horse, thereby conveying their own aplomb to the horse. The rider must give the horse enough time to realize that the unfamiliar object is not dangerous. If the horse tries to run away, the rider should not fight it unwisely, but quietly bring it to a halt and ride back without force to the same spot on a loose rein, until the horse realizes that there is no danger and behaves trustingly again. A horse which has been trained in this manner will later confidently go wherever the rider asks it to go; while at the same time remaining fully aware of its surroundings. It accurately registers every movement and any unfamiliar object in the distance by the direction of its gaze and the movement of its ears. In times of war, this ability has alerted riders on patrol to dangers which the human eye would not have been capable of seeing so early.

Through bad handling, impatience, and even punishment, shying can become a habitual vice which cannot be rectified any more by speaking calmly or by trying to get the horse used to many different objects. Such horses will shy repeatedly at unfamiliar objects. If they are securely on the aids, they cannot run away if they are ridden flexed to the outside past the source of fear, i.e., turned away in leg yield. Obedience to the aids must be stronger than the urge to shy, especially when the horse knows that the aids will be used very strongly and forcefully if it disobeys.

Horses must also learn to manage their own power. But they will never learn if they are not worked early on and frequently to the point of exhaustion. Horses which find canter exciting but are allowed to canter only for short distances, wear themselves out unnecessarily because they rush forward with all their power. However, if one makes a transition to canter after trotting steadily for several kilometers and rides along the same route in canter, the horses then learn to go at a steady canter and, especially important, develop a good breathing technique. These horses are powerful and able; they conserve energy in time and only use their full strength when the rider asks them to by means of strong driving aids.

It should always be clear to us that riding on an enclosed track and in the arena is a means to an end in the training of the riding horse which has become so firmly entrenched because up until now the greatest importance has been placed on dressage. If we consider obedience and training in open country to be of the same value, then we must also allow an equal amount of time while riding out. This is because obedience, dressage, and training must complement each other if the aim of training to produce an intelligent, obedient, agile, and lasting military horse is to be achieved.

Appendix

Position and Function of the Muscles

Only the muscles which are important for posture (carriage) and movement of the riding horse are included in this section. They have been grouped according to the parts of the body. However, some individual muscles have had to be dealt with in conjunction with other parts of the body as they are functionally connected to them.

The Muscles of the Neck and Upper Neck

The ***M. semispinalis capitis***, the **strong supporting muscle of the head**.

Broad point of origin: *Membrana dorsoscapularis* – the dorsoscapular membrane; the transverse processes of the first six to seven thoracic vertebrae as well as the articular processes of the last five cervical vertebrae.

Insertion: By means of a strong tendon on the squamous part of the occipital bone. The muscle is permeated by five strong tendinous strips which run at an angle to the fiber direction of the muscle fibrils. They divide the long muscle into successively arranged segments with short muscle fibers and, by doing so, increase the working power of the whole muscle which is thus capable of developing considerably more power and endurance.

Function: Suspending the head-neck lever on the withers in elastic tension. The muscle requires a long period of training to fulfill this function. This explains many of the neck problems of young horses which seek the contact with a lowered head well for a certain time, only to suddenly go with a raised head against the rein again. Fatigue of the *M. semispinalis* is the reason for this. Dismounting for a short time often makes any conflict with the rider superfluous; in most cases, the horse willingly accepts the contact again with a lowered head after a period of rest.

The ***M. longissimus cervicis***, the **long muscle of the neck**.

Origin: Transverse processes of the first six to seven thoracic vertebrae and the *Membrana dorsoscapularis*.

Insertion: 7th to 4th cervical vertebra. The external surface of its segments is overlaid with tendons; from the rear, its area of origin is covered with the tendinous extensions of the *Longissimus dorsi*.

Function: The *Longissimus cervicis* primarily has a static function. The cervical spine of the horse has an S-shape when the head is raised. In this position, the section from the 4th to 7th cervical vertebra toward the back is concave. The *Longissimus cervicis* inserts into this concave curve. When the neck is stretched in a low position it works in conjunction with the shoulders-withers sheet to suspend the neck on the withers.

As the muscle increases in size through training it carries out an active role. It raises the 4th to 7th cervical vertebra, whereby the concave curve stretches, the neck loses its S-shape, and a more attractive, even, and convex curve develops towards the back. The neck thereby becomes longer. Good riders often succeed in transforming the necks of young horses to a surprising extent by strengthening and increasing the size of the dorsal upper neck muscles, including the *M. serratus ventralis cervicis*, through training. On the other hand, incorrectly starting a young horse can turn the attractive neck of a riding horse into an ewe neck through atrophy and atony of these muscles. In this case, the sides of neck above the cervical spine display the large triangular indentation between the cervical spine, shoulder, and the crest of the mane.

The ***M. longissimus capitis*** and the ***M. longissimus atlantis***, the **long head muscle** (head and neck section).

Origin: Together with the *M. semispinalis capitis* on the transverse processes of the first two to three cervical vertebrae and the articular processes of the last five cervical vertebrae.

Insertion: Mastoid process of the temporal bone and the wing of the atlas.

Connected to the *M. splenius* by strong fleshy strips and the *M. brachiocephalicus* by a broad aponeurosis.

Function: Sideways movement of the head and neck; in equestrian terms: lateral bend while riding flexed to the left or right. In combination with the *Splenius* and brachiocephalic muscles its function is also dependent on the suppleness of these muscles, and they are all simultaneously connected to the rhythm of the movement. Unilateral contraction of the muscle makes the horse give to the increased pressure of the rein on this side. A characteristic of nearly all horses is that they bend the neck willingly to one side when the rein is applied unilaterally, while they resist the rein aid on the other side. On the basis of experience, 90% of horses stiffen the left side of the neck during training and bend willingly to the right, while becoming heavy on the left rein or going against it and avoiding the right rein by turning the head away, which makes them come behind the bit on the right side, i.e., they do not accept the bit. We therefore talk about the inborn bend to the right or "crookedness" of the horse, the cause of which is said to be the position of the foal in its mother's womb, but this has not been proven. In any case, straightness is one of the greatest obstacles to be overcome over the course of training of a horse and a large percentage of riders never attains even contact, but always has more weight on the left rein than on the right.

The M. splenius, the **spleen-shaped muscle**.

Origin: Top of the 2nd to 5th spines of the withers, *Membrana dorsoscapularis* and nuchal ligament.

Broad point of insertion:

1. on the transverse processes of the 5th to 3rd cervical vertebra,
2. on the tendon of the *M. longissimus atlantis*,
3. with the tendon of the *M. longissimus capitis* on the occipital bone.

The body of muscle is entirely fleshy, its insertion is partially aponeurotic. The *M. rhomboideus* and *M. serratus cervicalis* extend over the *M. splenius*. The *Splenius* forms an indented area between these muscles which narrows toward the withers. In horses with poorly developed upper neck muscles, this small triangular area is clearly visible in front of the withers. This "hole" disappears in correctly ridden horses as the *M. splenius* and *M. semispinalis* develop as a result of training and bulge outward.

Function: Sudden strong contractions of the *Splenius* and *M. semispinalis capitis* occasionally make the horse shake its head during training at which point the rider sees the nuchal ligament beneath the crest of the mane almost as a serpentine before them. The *M. splenius* should not function at all until the neck has attained its correct riding position by means of the other musculature of the upper neck (see Chapter 2) and is fixed on the withers. Its functions are the large movements of the neck which are necessary at a full gallop and to maintain balance across country or over obstacles. It works in the same direction as the *M. semispinalis capitis* which gives the neck its shape by "carrying it" while the *Splenius* serves to provide freedom of movement. This can only be effective in riding if the shape has been established when first starting a horse. Otherwise, it leads to an ewe neck and is followed invariably by the horse hollowing its back or working without its back.

The ***M. recti capitis dorsales*** **(major and minor)**, the **straight poll muscles** (large and small).

Origin: Crest and dorsal arc of the 2nd and 1st cervical vertebra.

Insertion: The squamous part of the occipital bone. They connect to the *M. semispinalis capitis* and have the same function. In elastic extension, they carry and suspend the head together with this muscle; their sudden jerky contraction leads to the shaking of the head.

The ***M. obliquus capitis caudalis***, the **oblique rear (caudal) muscle of the poll**.
Origin: Crest and dorsal side of the 2nd cervical vertebra.

Insertion: Upper side the frontal edge of the wing of the atlas.

Function: During bilateral contraction, it acts as a stabiliser. During unilateral contraction, it rotates the joint between the 1st and 2nd cervical vertebra. It is relatively strong and carries out the rotation of the head when it acts unilaterally. The oblique caudal muscle is covered by its own aponeurosis and superficially by the end-tendons of *Splenius* and *Brachiocephalic*. It is therefore also connected with the two main muscles. If this muscle is negatively tensed unilaterally, this leads to the so-called "tilting in the poll." The head is not bent sideways but rotated in the 2nd joint of the head, so that the rider sees one ear of the horse lower and the other higher. The cramped flexion of the neck to one side goes readily hand in hand with this position (see *Longissimus capitis* and *atlantis*) in which the neck displays a lateral kink between the 1st and 2nd cervical vertebra when seen from above. In the riding horse, an even bilateral coordination with the musculature of the upper neck is desirable.

The ***M. obliquus capitis cranialis***, the **oblique frontal muscle of the poll.**

Origin: Front edge and lower surface of the wing of the atlas.

Insertion: The sides of the back of the head.

Function: Extensor of the poll in the first joint of the head; used unilaterally it supports the *M. obliquus capitis caudalis.*

The ***Mm. recti capitis ventralis and lateralis***, the **short flexor muscles of the head.**

Origin: Ventral arch of the atlas.

Insertion: Base of the skull and the jugular process of the occipital bone.

Function: Flexors of the poll. Their activity is not desirable in riding; when they contract, the horse actively bends too much in the neck (hyper-flexion) and comes behind the bit.

The ***M. longus colli***, the **long deep flexor of the neck.**

Origin: Body of the 6th to 1st thoracic vertebra and body and transverse processes of the 7th to 3rd cervical vertebra.

Insertion: Body of the 7th to 1st cervical vertebra.

Function: For riding, it is of little importance, it acts as padding for the cervical spine, similar to the ***M. intertransversarii*** (muscles located between the vertebrae). It is, however, involved in all the movements of the spine as a result of its arrangement and it increases the stability of the cervical spine to cope with violent flexion. When this muscle is negatively tensed, it can make itself felt in an uncomfortable way by stiffening the spine. As the *M. longus colli* actively contracts, the horse "hyper-flexes" in the neck and, depending on its temperament, becomes heavy in the hand or behind the bit.

From the rider's point of view, one should aim for a passive state of the lower neck muscles, which means that the *M. longus colli* certainly plays a part in lowering and bending the neck; however, it never has to overcome any real resistance because the head and neck are suspended passively on the withers in a supple horse (Chapter 2). In correctly ridden horses, one can detect a consistent "disappearance" of the flexor muscles of the neck compared to the musculature of the upper neck and, therefore, the neck becomes thinner on the ventral side of the cervical spine.

The ***M. longus capitis***, the **long deep flexor muscle of the head**.

Origin: Lower (distal) surfaces of the transverse processes of the 6th to 3rd cervical vertebra.

Insertion: Base of the skull.

Function: In the correctly ridden horse, this muscle is hardly used. If it is incorrectly contracted, it produces "the false bend," meaning a strong bending of the neck between the 2nd and 3rd cervical vertebra in which a distinct break is visible in the crest of the mane above the 2nd cervical vertebra. Such horses tend to go behind the bit (Chapter 8).

The Superficial Muscles of the Throat Region.

M. sternothyreoideus, the **chest-larynx muscle**.

M. sternohyoideus, the **chest-hyoid muscle**.

Origin: Manubrium of the sternum (*Cartilago manubrii*).

Insertion: Thyroid cartilage of the larynx; the body of the hyoid bone.

M. omohyoideus, the **shoulder-hyoid muscle**.

Origin: Lower shoulder fascia.

Insertion: On the body of the hyoid bone together with the *M. sternohyoideus*. It joins closely with the *M. brachiocephalus* on the lower part of the neck.

M. sternomandibularis, the **sternomandibular muscle or chest-jaw muscle which nods the head**.

Origin: Manubrium of the sternum (*Cartilago manubrii*).

Insertion: Back edge of the lower jaw.

Function: The first three muscles mentioned pull the hyoid bone and larynx toward the chest. The sternomandibular muscle can pull the loose lower jaw downward and thus open the mouth. However, when the teeth are clenched together, it bends the head on both sides with stronger effect than the flexor muscles of the head.

These muscles play a primary role in the riding horse's evasion methods of soft rein contact. If they are held tightly in a state of contraction, the horse hyperflexes its head down behind the vertical, leans heavily on the bit, and does not yield to the asking rein. The teeth are thereby firmly clenched together and the horse cannot chew the bit. The larynx and the tongue may also be pulled back at the same time. In this case, a more or less audible intake of breath can be heard, which, on occasion, can be confused with the true whistling noise of the larynx. However, the characteristic whistling or roaring sound does not occur; rather, a slurping sound is produced which is frequently and suddenly interrupted for an instant by the swallowing reflex, usually at the precise moment when the sound is at its loudest.

In contrast to the true whistling of the larynx, this sound stops immediately after the horse halts. It generally stops completely once these horses have learned to relax these muscles over the course of training. Equine experts explain this sound simply by the horse lifting its tongue. Breathlessness caused in the same way during inhaling can occasionally be observed in humans who are not used to running when they take up a sport.

Another vice which is difficult to cure is rhythmic chewing and noisy playing with the bit in trot. It has not been resolved whether the close connection between the *M. omohyoideus* and brachiocephalic muscles and its origin in the shoulder are responsible or whether this is a reflex stimulated by their attendant nerves. In any case, this rhythmic activity only stops as the horse becomes supple, i.e., as the neck is stretched and the horse takes the contact; the chewing becomes quiet and independent from the movement.

Just as all the flexor muscles of the head and neck, the muscles mentioned above play only a passive role in the carriage and movement of the riding horse. They should always be ready to yield and stretch. The horse which is correctly on the bit should be stretching into the contact with a rider's giving hand. If these muscles are not actively used, an increase in their size during training will never be observed, and the jugular groove becomes even more clearly defined on the well-developed neck of a riding horse.

The Muscles of the Back

The ***M. rhomboideus***, the **diamond-shaped muscle**.

Origin: Nuchal ligament from the level of the 2nd cervical vertebra down to the withers and to the protuberance of the 2nd to 8th (9th) spines of the withers; there it connects with the *M. dorsoscapularis*.

Insertion: Scapular cartilage. The *M. rhomboideus dorsi*, the rear (caudal) section of the diamond-shaped muscle (*Trapezius*), fills the space between the main lamella of the *Membrana dorsoscapularis* and the scapular cartilage up to the ends of the spinal processes of the vertebrae of the withers; it is, in effect, padding.

The *M. rhomboideus cervicis*, the neck section of the diamond-shaped muscle, extends from the front part of the lower surface of the scapular cartilage to the nuchal ligament; it moves the neck upward; in its passive role, it serves to transfer the movements of the forehand onto the poll (nodding movement in the rhythm of movement).

The ***Membrana dorsoscapularis***, the **withers-shoulder sheet.**

Together with the *M. rhomboideus* and *M. trapezius dorsi*, it connects the spines of the withers with the dorsal section of the shoulder blade and the ribs which lie below it; it also sinks in the form of a deep blade between the back muscles to the transverse processes of the vertebrae of the withers.

It forms the point of origin for the three muscles of the upper neck: *M. splenius, M. longissimus cervicis,* and *M. serratus semispinalis capitis* as well as for the *M. rhomboideus dorsi* and *M. serratus dorsalis cranialis.*

Function: By means of its attachment to the top of the spines of the withers, it transfers the pull of the muscles of the upper neck onto the withers; on the other hand, it forms the base on which the passive upper neck muscles are suspended. It transfers the movements generated by the shoulder in the form of swinging motions to the spine of the back as well as to the muscles of the upper neck.

The ***M. multifidus dorsi et lumborum***, the **multi-serrate muscle of the back and loins**.

Origin: In a row on all the spinous processes from the 7th cervical vertebra up to the last lumbar vertebra.

Insertion: In a row on the transverse or mammillary processes of the thoracic and lumbar vertebrae to the sacrum.

The muscle is composed of many strips of muscle, each one of which is covered by a flat tendon which strengthens it. It runs in a direction from the top front to the bottom at the back, whereby each strip of muscle skips two to six (seven) vertebrae. At the spinous processes of the withers, the muscle strips do not extend from the summits on which the pull of the upper neck muscles acts from the front, but rather from approximately half-way up the spinous processes. By these means, the upper neck muscles work on a much longer and, therefore, much more efficient lever arm, compared to the *M. multifidus*. The length of the spinous processes is proportional to the length and angle of the muscle strips; at the front they are longer and at a smaller angle, at the back shorter and steeper (Figure 4, see Page 33).

Function: The *M. multifidus* is suited to carry out static functions as a result of its tendinous reinforcements. It transfers the forward pull exerted by the upper neck muscles on its base, the spinous processes, in part directly and in part indirectly by means of the withers-shoulder sheet onto the vertebral bodies and thus prevents the back sagging downward. The *M. multifidus* acts as a strong elastic suspensory ligament. As such it also transfers the swinging movements in the rhythm of the movement of the forehand generated from the withers-shoulder sheet on the withers onto the back. The back thus receives the suppleness its needs to work correctly.

In a state of cramped contraction, the dorsal vertebrae would be pressed against each other and the back would become stiff – in equestrian terms, the horse's back would be tense; the rider sits as if on a hard wooden board.

The **lateral levator muscle of the tail** is the immediate continuation of the *M. multifidus*. In a supple back, it works in the same tensile direction as the multifidus muscle, hence, forward-upward, and, thus, carries the tail. A well-carried and evenly swinging tail is one of the indications for the trainer that the horse's back is supple.

The ***M. longissimus dorsi***, the **long muscle of the back.**
Two rows of origin, two rows of insertion.
Origin: Medial: First sacral vertebrae to 13th thoracic vertebra on the summits of the spinous processes; lateral: crest of the ilium (*Crista iliaca*) and its aponeurosis.
Insertion: Medial: *Processus mamillares* and *transversi* of the lumbar and thoracic vertebrae up to the 7th cervical vertebra; the attachments are tendinous; lateral: in the form of transverse sheets on all the ribs up to the 4th.
The muscle tapers to a tip from the 13th thoracic spinous processes to the 7th cervical vertebra. The direction of the fibers runs from top hind to bottom front. Toward the front, the muscle merges into flat tendons which belong to the medial row of insertion and insert into the first thoracic vertebrae and the 7th cervical vertebra; they extend across the *Longissimus cervicis.*

The ***superficial fascia*** of the ***M. longissimus dorsi***
is extremely strong, originates from the spines of the sacrum and the lumbar vertebrae and from the sacral tuberosity to the coxal tuberosity on the ilium. It merges with the fascia of the other side and disappears on the tip of the *Longissimus.* On the loins, it extends over the hollow of the muscle in which the lumbar head of the large gluteal muscle is attached.

Function: The long muscle of the back is mostly fleshy, therefore, it exerts only continuous contraction, i.e. is not suited to carrying weight. If it were spasmodically contracted, the result would be a stiffening of the back, but also premature fatigue. The long muscle of the back functions predominantly in canter to lift the forehand, during the course of which it contracts from its rear point of origin in the rhythm of the movement; this is especially the case during the canter take-off. It is well-known that frequent transitions between trot and canter encourage the activity of the back and also muscle development in weak backs. The long muscle of the back is connected to the large gluteal muscle by means of its fascia and, therefore, its work is integrally linked to and dependent on the rhythm of the movements of the hindquarters.
Its point of insertion on the ribs results in the ribs being held taut toward the back as long as the *Longissimus dorsi* is in a cramped state of tension. Only when this muscle is supple can the horse inhale freely.
The front section of the ***M. serratus dorsalis***, the ***rear section of the upper serrated muscle***, supports the *Mm. intercostales externi* as inspiratory muscles. It emanates from the deep sheet of the *Fascia lumbodorsalis* and the middle sheet of the *Membrana dorsoscapularis*. It is thus linked to the movement of the large muscles of the back and upper neck; its state of tension is influenced by these muscles. When the muscles of the back are tense, the front serrate section is also tense; but this hampers breathing. Conversely, supple back musculature allows the horse to breathe freely. This explains the observation that horses take quiet, deep breaths in the same moment that they begin to supple (see also *M. longissimus dorsi*) and audibly snort

as they exhale. Every rider knows that a horse which is breathing freely and snorts has now also relaxed its back and lets the rider sit comfortably without bouncing.

The ***M. latissimus dorsi***, the **broad muscle of the back**.

Origin: Out of the *Fascia lumbodorsalis* and through these connected to the spinous processes of the 3rd thoracic to the last lumbar vertebra.

Insertion: By a tendon medially on the proximal third of the humerus.

Function: It retracts the limbs, i.e., it pulls the distal part of the shoulder and the point of the shoulder back. In so doing, it acts low on the shoulder blade in the same direction of movement as the *M. serratus ventralis* acts above. Just like this muscle, the *M. latissimus dorsi* is placed under maximum strain, when the forehand pushes off from the ground and when the rotational movement of the shoulder is compressed during landing after a jump. Otherwise, it acts as the antagonist of the *M. brachiocephalicus*. When the back is tense, its connection to the *Fascia lumbodorsalis* inhibits the shoulder going forward – the so-called freedom of the shoulder. These horses then walk with short and choppy steps.

The largest (fleshy) section of the *M. latissimus dorsi* lies directly behind the shoulder musculature. If the muscle is still under-developed in younger horses, they do not yet have the conformation to position the saddle properly; this improves through progressive muscle growth during training.

The ***M. spinalis (et semispinalis dorsi et cervicis)***, the **withers muscle**.

It covers the spines of the withers laterally across the *M. multifidus* up to their summits, hence, it acts as padding there and extends over to the rear half of the neck. In the horse, it is composed of two sections, as its full name signifies, a back and a neck portion, of which one covers the other as far as both are positioned on the withers.

Back section:

Origin: Ends of the spinous processes of the lumbar vertebrae and the outer surface of the *Longissimus dorsi* covered by fascia.

Insertion: Ends of the spinous processes of the 7th to 1st thoracic vertebra.

Neck section:

Origin: Lateral surfaces of the ends of half of the spinous processes in the withers area.

Insertion: Spinous process of the 7th to 3rd cervical vertebra.

Function: It supports the head as does *M. longissimus cervicis* and transfers the movement of the neck over the withers onto the long muscle of the back and vice versa.

The ***M. trapezius thoracis***, the **top of the withers muscle**, a relatively thick, triangular muscle in the rear withers area.

Origin: Withers section of the nuchal ligament and 3rd to 12th spinous process of the thoracic spine, partially covered by the *Fascia lumbodorsalis*.

Insertion: Scapular spine up to the supraglenoid tubercle. Its aponeurosis becomes the shoulder-arm fascia (*Fascia omobrachialis*) and the general fascia of the upper neck (*Fascia colli*).

Function: Extends the limbs forward and lifts the distal parts of the shoulder away from the torso in the lateral movements. Furthermore, it is important padding for the area on which to position the saddle on a horse.

The Muscles of the Forehand

The ***M. brachiocephalicus***, the **head-neck-arm muscle**.

Origin:

1. on the temporal bone and with the tendon of the *M. longissimus capitis* and splenius on the occipital bone,
2. on the tendon of the *M. longissimus atlantis*,
3. on the 2nd to 4th cervical vertebra.

Insertion: Front surface of the humerus and fascia of the lower arm (together with the *M. pectoralis humeri descendens*).
The neck fascia is inserted on the upper neck edge of the muscle. The brachiocephalic muscle is connected with the *Splenius* over a broad area at its points of origin on the head and neck.

Function: The *M. brachiocephalicus* swings the front leg forward. Its tensile direction runs approximately parallel to the cervical spine. For this reason, the movement of the forehand is dependent on the position of the neck. During racing, the action of the forehand is flat and ground-covering with the neck stretched far out but straight forward, however, with a strongly raised neck, it is high and covers little ground ("knee action"). A neck which is short in itself, whether it is tightened in the form of an ewe neck or whether it is hyper-flexed, shortens the range of action of the head-neck-arm muscle and, thus, the ground coverage of the front leg. The movement can only become elevated **and** ground-covering when the neck attains the perfect shape for riding which combines the greatest possible stretching and relative elevation.
The joint point of origin of the *Brachiocephalicus* and *Splenius* is of great importance for maintaining balance and, thus, sure-footedness across country. When the horse stumbles on uneven terrain or after a jump, it can only bring the front leg which is stopping the fall and, thus, saving horse and rider far forward if it can stretch its neck (not lift it!; see *M. splenius*). If the rider is leaning on the reins or even tries to pull the horse's head up, this hinders the horse's natural reaction and the stumble is usually followed by a fall.
These interrelations make it especially clear why freedom in the shoulder is dependent on the suppleness of the musculature of the upper neck.

The ***M. serratus ventralis cervicis***, the **neck section of the lower serrated muscle.**

Origin: Medial surface of the shoulder blade close to the base (front section).

Insertion: Transverse processes of the 7th to 4th cervical vertebra.

Function: It is a compact fleshy mass, not inlaid with tendons and not covered by the *Fascia serrata*, but very strong. It is one of the most active movement muscles of the shoulder. On the one hand, it pulls the dorsal section of the shoulder forward and acts by contracting strongly when the forehand swings or pushes off from the ground in the extended gaits and, above all, during a jump; on the other hand, it takes the initial weight as the horse lands after a jump, whereby it stops an excessively strong rotation, i.e., a steeply angled position of the shoulder. The trained jumping horse lands with its neck stretched far forward. In this position, the muscle is stretched, which increases its strength and reduces the reaction time. Such a horse can already push off with the forehand during the moment of landing; it remains in movement and does not lose any time. In contrast, horses which land with a high neck, always pause in their movement, lose time, and require split seconds to prepare themselves for the next canter stride. Old jumping horses display an enormous increase in the size of the *M. serratus ventralis cervicis* through training; the muscle bulges in front of the shoulder blade and, at rest, the shoulder is positioned at a steeper angle by the tonus (the natural tension) of the muscle. Consequently, the forehand is camped under.

The ***M. scalenus primae costae***, the **suspensory muscle of the ribs**.

Origin: Upper 2/3rds of the 1st rib.

Insertion: Transverse processes of the 7th to 4th cervical vertebra.

Function: The muscle is not tendinous, but very strong. If it contracts with a raised neck from its point of origin, the 1st rib, it makes the caudal section of the neck sag downward and, with the simultaneous action of the upper neck muscles, causes the undesirable S-form of the cervical spine, i.e., the ewe neck. In horses which have worked with an ewe neck for their whole life, one can observe large bundles of muscles in this area as a result of hypertrophy (enlargement) of the *M. scalenus*. It is out of the question that this purely fleshy muscle ventral to the cervical spine secures the neck into position on the withers as this would be synonymous with "restraining" the neck. It is even more improbable, according to the theory of the "muscle ring" (**Simon, Haase**) that the muscle suspends the ribs with the neck fixed in a certain position, i.e., it holds the thoracic cage in a forward position on the 1st rib and, thus, indirectly becomes an antagonist of the straight abdominal muscle. It is certainly not strong enough to carry out such a feat of strength, and the flexible cervical spine would not be suitable as a base of action in comparison to stability of the thorax.
The *M. scalenus* works unilaterally when the neck is bent to the side. Its main function is in conjunction with the *M. serratus ventralis cervicis*. When this

muscle is placed under maximum strain, the scalene muscle works together with it by anchoring this pull on the cervical spine onto the thorax. The hypertrophy developed through work of the *M. scalenus* together with that of the *M. serratus ventralis cervicis* can almost always be observed in experienced old jumping horses, steeplechasers, and racehorses; conversely, it cannot be seen so clearly in riding school horses.

The ***M. supraspinatus***, the **muscle of the cranial part of the scapular spine**.

Origin: In the entire rim of the *Fossa supraspinata*.

Insertion: With two branches on both, the greater and lesser tubercles on the proximal end of the upper arm, to both sides of the groove for the biceps origin tendon (*Sulcus intertubercularis*).
It fills the *Fossa supraspinata* of the shoulder blade and continues forward over the shoulder joint by splitting into two branches which allow the *M. biceps* to pass between them.

Function: Extensor of the shoulder joint, holds the shoulder joint as the shock is absorbed after a jump. It is especially well defined in jumping horses.

The ***M. biceps brachii***, the **straight flexor of the elbow**.

Origin: On the *Tuberositas supraglenoidalis*, a dent on the distal end of the neck edge of the *Scapula*.

Insertion: *Tuberositas radii*, medial at the front on the proximal end of the radius.

It forms a fleshy body which is nevertheless strong, and which does not stick out during contraction as a bulbous bulge on the upper arm as in humans, because it is much too strongly inlaid with tendons and covered by the brachiocephalic muscle. It extends down the neck at the front over the shoulder joint and also down in front of the humerus in such a manner that it passes medially in front of the elbow joint and terminates on the *Tuberculum radii*.
From its origin to below the *Sulcus intertubercularis* it is practically entirely tendinous; at this point it has a deep groove into which the *Tuberculum intermedium* fastens like a button in a loop in a standing horse. And from this point, the muscle, which is composed of oblique fibers, allows a flat, superficial, very strong strip of tendon to reach the end-tendon. From this strip, a tight, flat strip of tendon, the *Lacertus fibrosus*, branches off close to the elbow joint and, easily palpable, bypasses laterally at the front the groove between the humerus and forearm musculature. Having continued over the rounded surface of the *M. extensor carpi radialis (M. radialis dorsalis)*, it terminates with its end-tendon on the protuberance of the fore cannon bone (3rd metacarpal bone). This is why this tendon is called *Tendo metacarpi* of the *Biceps brachii*.

Function: The *M. biceps* is a tireless supporting belt which is stretched in front of the shoulder joint and stops it from giving way, however, under the condition, that the elbow joint is fixed in place and the attachment of the biceps is fixed on the

Tuberositas radii. At the same time, the biceps belt causes the shoulder and elbow joints to be tied together in flexion in such a manner that the one cannot be bent without the other.

The tendon of the biceps (*Lacertus fibrosus*) transfers its tension onto the carpal joint ("knee"). Conversely, the biceps belt is contracted as this joint is flexed, whereby the shoulder joint is stretched. On the strongly flexed leg, which is placed on the ground, as is the case for example during a stumble or the beginning of a fall, this construction automatically exerts a pull on the *M. biceps* and, thus, stretches the shoulder joint; therefore, it contributes to helping the horse to rise in the forehand.

The ***Mm. anconaei***, the **extensor muscles of the elbow**.

Origin: The *Caput longum* on the caudal rim of the shoulder blade, the *Caput laterale* and *mediale* on the lateral and medial longitudinal ridge of the humerus.

Insertion: Protuberance of the elbow, *Tuber olecrani.*

Function: They converge from the long line of origin on the shoulder blade and humerus onto the process of the elbow, fill the triangular space between the shoulder blade and the humerus and form a cushion-like layer on the side of the chest wall, which should be as well-defined as possible. These muscles are relaxed in the standing horse. The theory that they maintain a labile balance of the elbow joint by pulling on the point of the elbow and, thus, enable the horse to stand without tiring is incorrect. The lack of any tendinous inlay does not permit the hypothesis of a static function. The *Mm. anconaei* have two completely opposite functions, as do the buttock muscles. During the initial phase of movement, they are the flexors of the shoulder joint of the swinging leg by means of the pull on the point of the elbow; conversely, on the supporting leg, this pull on the point of the elbow works to extend the elbow joint and this action is transferred onto the shoulder joint via the supporting belt of the biceps. The collaboration with the *M. serratus ventralis cervicis* is imperative for this function. The *Mm. anconaei* extend the elbow joint as the front leg supports and pushes off; but they can only do this if the shoulder blade is held predominantly at a steep angle by the *M. serratus cervicis.*

As the neck is stretched down, the action of both muscles is transferred forward; the muscles themselves are stretched and can act with maximum strength out of this position. These interactions are a further explanation for why the horse should land after a jump with its neck down and not raised.

The Flexor Muscles of the Toe

The ***M. flexor digitalis profundus***, the **deep flexor muscle of the toe or deep digital flexor tendon**, is a muscle composed of three heads, of which the most important one originates on the medial epicondyle (flexor) of the humerus at the back above the elbow joint. This head is split again into three branches which are all strongly inlaid with tendons and made up of short muscle fibers which run in an oblique direction. It runs down the back of the lower arm against the carpal joint, where it merges with the two other muscle heads to form the strong deep flexor tendon. Half-way down the metacarpal bone this acquires the extremely strong *Caput tendineum*, supporting or carpal check ligament, which emerges from the volar bundle of ligaments of the carpal bone.

Origin: *Epicondylus flexorius* of the humerus.

Insertion: *Facies flexoria* of the coffin bone (distal phalanx).

The ***M. flexor digitalis superficialis***, the **superficial flexor muscle of the toe or superficial digital flexor tendon**, is a single muscle which runs along the lower arm next to the deep digital flexor muscle. Its tendon is, however, positioned superficially behind the tendon of the deep digital flexor muscle. It also has a *Caput tendineum*, a supporting or radial check ligament, which originates from the middle part of the rear surface of the radius and already meets the tendon above the carpal bone.

Origin: *Epicondylus flexorius* of the humerus.

Insertion: With two branches on the flexor tuberosity of the short pastern bone (middle phalanx).

The **suspensory ligament** functions autonomously, is composed of the entirely tendinous ***M. interosseous medius***, the **provimal sesamoid bones (fetlock joint)**, and the **distal ligaments** of the **proximal sesamoid bones** (*Ligament sesamoideum rectum* and *Ligament sesamoidea obliqua*).

In literature, the upper sesamoideum ligament, which is the purely tendinous medial interosseus muscle, is placed facing the lower sesamoideum ligaments.

Function: The end sections of the tendons of both digital flexors, each with a check ligament, and the suspensory ligament are supporting belts positioned overlapping across the back of the fetlock joint. These supporting belts are tensed to support as the joint is overextended and have to hold the joint. However, the consonance in the function of these three components does not stand up to closer inspection. The statistics of injuries of tendons and ligaments teaches us otherwise. The riding horse, and especially the racehorse, primarily develop conditions of the superficial digital flexor tendon and occasionally of the suspensory ligament, while inflammations of the deep digital flexor tendon in horses that pull heavy loads is the rule. The reason for this is to be found in the fact that the three sections of this suspensory apparatus reach down to different levels on the toe and race- and draught horses place maximum strain in different ways on their phalangeal joints during the phases of movement. In the racehorse, the passive stay apparatus is subjected to maximum strain during the supporting phase and especially in the moment the leg supports the weight (at its greatest at full gallop and above all during landing after a jump), that is as the fetlock joint is sagging, but as the coffin joint is bent (volar-flexed). In the draught horse, however, this apparatus is stretched to the maximum in the moment of pushing off from the ground, whereby the fetlock and pastern joints are held in the middle position, the coffin joint, however, is in maximum dorsal flexion. Therefore, in racehorses the superficial digital flexor tendon and the suspensory ligament are stretched to the maximum as the weight is taken on the leg because they only extend to the pastern and the proximal and middle phalanges; the deep digital flexor tendon is, however, relatively relaxed, as it also extends over and beyond the coffin joint during its flexion. In the draught horse, only the deep digital flexor tendon is placed under great strain as it pushes off from the ground, because in this moment the superficial digital flexor tendon and suspensory ligament are relatively relaxed because of the extended position of both proximal (upper) phalangeal joints.

The strongly tendinous muscles are the extensor or supporting muscles of the elbow joint on the supporting leg; as tendinous ligament structures, they stop it from buckling as weight is placed on it.

The Muscles of the Chest

The ***M. serratus ventralis thoracis***, the **lower serrated muscle, suspensory muscle of the torso**.

Origin: Medial surface of the shoulder blade close to the base (caudal section).

Insertion: Fan-shaped with strips of muscle with jagged ends on the 1st to 9th rib (supporting ribs!).

Reinforcement:

1. by means of a large amount of tendinous inlay,
2. by means of the very strong *Fascia serrata* which covers the outside of the muscle, attaches to the lower rim of the area of origin on the ribs, and extends in the form of the *Tunica flava* across the oblique external abdominal muscle to the ventral middle line of the thorax, where it joins the other side.

The *M. serratus* is inlaid with 12 to 20 strips (*Lamina superficialis*), branching off the withers-shoulder sheet, which enter on its medial surface and insert on the *Fascies serrata* of the shoulder blade.

Function: Suspensory muscle of the torso. The thorax is elastically suspended between both shoulder blades.

The four ***Mm. pectorales***, the **muscles of the chest**, of which the 1st and 2nd belong to the *M. pectoralis profundus* (deep pectoral muscle) but the 3rd and 4th to the *M. pectoralis superficialis*, the superficial pectoral muscle.

The ***M. pectoralis praescapularis***, the **chest-shoulder muscle**.

Origin: On the sternum from the point of attachment of the 4th to 1st rib.

Insertion: Pulling obliquely upward on the neck edge of the shoulder blade.

The ***M. pectoralis humeri ascendens***, the **deep chest-humerus muscle**.

Origin: On the sternum from the point of attachment of the 4th to 8th rib and on the *Tunica flava* in the area of and behind the xiphoid cartilage.

Insertion: On the upper end of the humerus (on the tubercles of the longitudinal groove).

Function: Suspensory muscles of the torso. They also pull the point of the shoulder back and prevent overly excessive flexion of the shoulder during landing after a jump. Together with the *Latissimus dorsi*, they are the antagonists of the *Brachiocephalicus*.

The ***M. pectoralis humeri descendens***, the **superficial chest-humerus muscle**.

Origin: On the ridge of the *Manubrium sterni*.

Insertion: Pulls obliquely downward and toward the rear, on the front surface of the humerus and on the upper arm fascia.

The ***M. pectoralis transversus***, the **underarm sheet of the chest muscle**.

Origin: On *Crista sterni* (sternum), in the region of the 1st to 6th rib; the muscles of both sides are connected together along the middle line of the body.

Insertion: Medial section of the forearm fascia close to the elbow joint.

Function: Pulls the forelimbs inward; the *M. pectoralis humeri descendants* also moves the swinging leg forward.

The Muscles of the Hindquarters

The Gluteal Muscles

The ***M. glutaeus profundus***, the **deep muscle of the gluteal area**.

Origin: *Spina ischiadica* of the pelvis

Insertion: *Trochanter major anterior*, upper edge.

The ***M. glutaeus medius***, the **large or middle muscle of the gluteal area**.
Its deep section: the *M. glutaeus accessorius*.

Origin: Wing of the ilium from the hip joint to the sacral tuberosity, 1st and 2nd spinous processes of sacrum; with the lumbar spur on the fascia of the long muscle of the back.
The *M. glutaeus accessorius*: lateral half of the wing of the ilium up to the *Linea glutaea*.

Insertion: The *M. glutaeus accessorius* inserts distally to the *Trochanter major anterior* after crossing it; the superficial main section with a large tendon on the *Trochanter major posterior*, which extends in the form of a lever arm far over the ball joint of the hip. Its fleshy part also inserts over and beyond the trochanter on the caudal surface of the *Os femoris (M. piriformis)*.

Function: It is the extensor of the hip joint during pushing off and together with the *Longissimus dorsi* lifts the forehand during a transition to canter.
As the extensor muscle of the hip joint, it maintains the flexion of this joint as the haunches flex (Chapter 4). Its lumbar origin extends over the entire back of the lumbar region to the front. Its coupling with the *Longissimus dorsi* forces the musculature of the back and gluteal area to work in the same rhythm.

The ***M. glutaeus superficialis***, the **superficial muscle of the gluteal area**.

Origin: By means of the gluteal fascia on the *Tuber coxae* and the 2nd sacral spinous process.

Insertion: *Trochanter tertius femoris*. It is closely joined to the *M. tensor fasciae latae* which has the same function.

Function: As opposed to the other gluteal muscles, it is the flexor of the hip joint on the supporting leg.

The Inner Lumbar Muscles

The ***M. psoas minor***, the **small lumbar muscle**.

Origin: Medial to the *Psoas major* on the bodies of the last three thoracic vertebrae and of the first four lumbar vertebrae.

Insertion: *Tuberculum psoadicum* of the body of the ilium.

Function: To place the pelvis at a steep angle (during urination or coitus).

The ***M. iliopsas*** comprised of the **double-headed *M. iliacus*** and the ***M. psoas major***.

The ***M. iliacus***, the **muscle of the ilium**.

Origin: *Fossa muscularis* of the body of the ilium, wing of the sacrum, and the front surface of the wings of the ilium.

Insertion: With the tendon of the *Psoas major* on the *Trochanter minor femoris*.

The ***M. psoas major***, the **large lumbar muscle**.

Origin: On the 17th and 18th rib and the transverse processes of the first five lumbar vertebrae.

Insertion: *Trochanter minor femoris* (medial side of the femur or bone).

Function: The *M. iliopsoas* is the flexor of the hip joint.

The Long Muscles of the Ischium

The **long muscles of the ischium** are the *M. biceps femoris*, the *M. semitendinosus*, and the *M. semimembranosus*.

The biceps lies laterally on the croup and femur for its entire length. The *Semitendinosus* and *Semimembranosus* cross onto the medial side on the femur. Together, they form the buttocks. Each of these muscles has a vertebral and ischiatic head.

The ***M. biceps femoris***, the **lateral (outer) long muscle of the ischium.**
It is one of the strongest individual muscles of the body.

Origin: Vertebral head: spinal process of the 2nd to 4th of the sacral vertebra.
Ischiatic head: dorsal on the lateral surface of the ischial tuberosity.

Insertion: On the rear surface of the *Os femoris* close to the *Trochanter tertius* and the lateral side of the stifle; there it forms three branches: 1st to the patella, 2nd to the *Ligament rectunt patellae laterale* (lateral straight patellar ligament) and to the *Tuberositas tibiae*; the 3rd phases out in the form of the *Tendo accessorius* to the *Tuber calcanei* and into the *Fascia cruris* (fascia of the lower limb).

The ***M. semitendinosus***, the **caudal (rear) long muscle of the ischium.**

Origin: Vertebral head: on the spinal process of the 5th sacral vertebra and the first two coccygeal vertebrae.
Ischiatic head: lateral on the ventral surface of the ischial tuberosity.

Insertion: With two branches, 1. medial with its tendon on the *Crista tibiae*, 2. its aponeurosis forms the *Tendo accessorius*, which goes to the *Tuber calcanei*; otherwise, it radiates to the *Fascia cruris*.

The ***M. semimembranosus***, the **medial (inner) long muscle of the ischium.**

Origin: Vertebral head: rear edge of the broad pelvic ligament and on the 1st coccygeal vertebra; the latter in attachment with an aponeurosis with the *M. semitendinosus.*

Ischiatic head: medial on the ventral surface of the ischial tuberosity. If it is well developed, the cleft between the thighs when viewed from behind is narrow.

Insertion: *Epicondylus medialis femoris* and the medial collateral ligament of the stifle joint; it therefore remains above the stifle and is shorter than the other ischiatic muscles. It corresponds approximately to the cranial branch of the *Biceps femoris* on the lateral side. All three long muscles of the ischium are essentially fleshy.

Function: The *Biceps* and *Semitendinosus* are flexors of the stifle joint on the swinging leg. However, on the supporting leg, all three muscles together are extensors of the hip and stifle joints in the push-off phase, as well as the hock joint, in that they pull the angle of the stifle rearward and extend the joint of the hock by means of the pull of their accessory ligaments onto the calcaneal tuberosity. Otherwise, the stifle and hock joints are interdependent as a result of the tendinous brace of the *Tendo femoro tarseus* in front of and the large *Achilles tendon* behind the *tibia* (see below). As the extensor muscles keep the appropriate joints on the leg which is taking the weight flexed, that is to say, prevent it from giving way to any greater degree, the *Biceps, Semitendinosus* and *Semimembranosus* support the flexion of the stifle and hock joints, and, hence, the hip joint, as the haunches are flexed. As these muscles increase in size as a result of training, the round shape of the buttocks becomes more clearly defined, and both of the inner surfaces of the thighs come into contact with each other over a greater area in the cleft between the thighs than is the case in young horses. When such horses sweat, white foam forms in the cleft between the thighs as a result of the skin rubbing. If this cleft between the thighs is narrow in a young horse, the muscles are naturally pre-disposed, and the rider can conclude from this that such horses are especially suitable for dressage. One can only learn to judge this through the experience gained by comparison.

The Front (Cranial) Femur Muscles

The ***M. quadriceps femoris***, the **extensor muscle of the patella**.

Origin: On the body of the ilium close to the acetabulum and on the front and side surfaces of the femur.

Insertion: On the patella and by means of the straight patellar ligaments on the tibial tuberosity.

The ***M. tensor fascia latae***, the **tensor muscle of the fascia of the femur**.

Origin: Coxal tuberosity.

Insertion: Its aponeurosis becomes the *Fascia lata* and *genus* and attaches to the patella.

Function: During pushing off from the ground, they act as extensors of the stifle joint, and on the swinging leg, a section (*M. rectus femoris*) acts as flexor of the hip joint. During flexion of the haunches, and generally in the supporting phase, the *Quadriceps femoris* acts as a support to the patella. If it is paralyzed (hemoglobinuria), the horse's hind leg gives way during the supporting phase because it cannot support the weight of the body. The fleshy but powerful extensor of the patella is therefore substantially involved in flexing the haunches. The lack of tendinous reinforcement results in early fatigue and presents the rider with problems in the hindquarters. Training this group of muscles must be carried out especially carefully and consistently.

The Tendon Brace Between the Stifle and Hock Joint

Two tendon apparatuses are stretched from the femur to the *Tarso-metatarsus* (the tarsal and metatarsal bones of the horse are effectively joined together in an immobile unit): one simple apparatus which extends down in front of the tibia, called the *Tendo femoro tarseus* (flexor of the hock, part of the stay apparatus) and one complex structure, the *Tendo communis calcis* (strong distal tendon of the muscles on the caudal part of the hind limbs), which accompanies the *Tibia* on the rear (plantar) side.

The ***Tendo femoro tarseus*****, (flexor of the hock, part of the stay apparatus)** denoted by some authors as the *M. peronaeus tertius*, is an entirely tendinous cord as thick as a finger.

Origin: *Fossa muscularis*, at the distal end of the femur, close beneath the lateral trocheal reach.

Insertion: In three end beams which, together with the two end-tendons of the *M. tibialis anterior*, encircle the *tarsus* and the proximal end of the metatarsal bones from the front and side.

The ***Tendo communis calcis*****, common calcaneal tendon** is the thick tendon cord which extends down from the calf to the calcaneal tuberosity (point of the hock) and is composed of three different individual structures: *Tendo plantaris, Tendo calcaneus,* and *Tendo accesssorius.*

1. The ***Tendo plantaris*** is the proximal section of the superficial digital flexor tendons of the middle phalanx, *M. flexor digitalis pedis superficialis* which extends from the femur to the calcaneal tuberosity The muscle belly, which is contained by the muscles of the gaskin, has very little muscle as a result of tendinous restructuring and is only slightly stronger than its tendon section, which is barely the thickness of a thumb: in practice, it can only be considered as a passively acting tendinous ligament structure.

Origin: *Fossa plantaris* of the femur.

Insertion: On the calcaneal tuberosity as the tendon which descends to the flexor tuberosity of the middle phalanx (the superficial digital flexor tendon) spreads out like a cap on the calcaneal tuberosity and the edges of this cap fuse strongly with the protuberance of the hock.

Function of the *Tendo femoro tarseus* and *Tendo plantaris*: To fix the tibia between the femur and the *Tarso-metatarsus* and to automatically place the stifle and hock joints in a state of interdependence. These are therefore braced together in flexion as well as extension by means of the two tendon cords in such a way that flexion and extension of the stifle initiate the same movements in the hock joint and vice versa. Both of these tendinous ligament structures are important for the flexion of the haunches, during which, by means of the action of the long ischiadic muscles, the patella is held in elastic flexion, which automatically transfers itself onto the hock joint.

2. The ***Tendo calcaneus***, is the tendon apparatus of the three-headed calf muscle, the *M. triceps surae*. It is composed of the *Tendo gastrocnemius* and *Tendo soleus*. The ***Tendo gastrocnemius*** is the tendon of the calf muscle (of the same name), also called the achilles tendon. It winds itself lengthwise in a half spiral twist around the *Tendo plantaris* to then attach itself onto the calcaneal tuberosity beneath the plantar tendon.

The ***Tendo soleus*** (*Tendo femoro calcaneus*) is a flat tendon cord connected to the weak *M. soleus*.

Origin: With the lateral *Gastrocnemius*, which it lies closely against, on the femur laterally next to the *Fossa plantaris*.

Insertion: With the *Tendo accessorius* (see below), which originates from the *Biceps* and *Semitendinosus*, running down in front of the *Tendo plantaris* and *Tendo calcaneus* on the calcaneal tuberosity. The *M. soleus* sinks in a hand's width above the *Tuber calcanei*.

Function: Supports the *Tendo plantaris* in bracing the tibia in flexed gait.

3. The ***Tendo accessorius*** is a tendon cord which it is not possible to distinguish clearly from the fascia of the calf and which is formed laterally by means of the common calcaneal tendon of the *Biceps* and medially by means of the tendon of the *Semitendinosus*. These two meet head-on with the Achilles and plantar tendon and form a single unit with the laterally descending *Tendo soleus*, which extends down to the calcaneal tuberosity.

Insertion: On the front edge of the *Tuber calcanei* and, encircling it to both sides, on the insertion of the cap on the hock.

Function: To transfer the extending action of the *Biceps* and *Semitendinosus* onto the hock joint and to support the bracing of the tibia in the flexed gait. Thus, the true extensor of the foot joint, the *M. triceps surae*, receives two strong direct assistants which are lacking in humans. And all the supporters and extensors of the stifle indirectly become assistants of the extensor of the foot.

The Abdominal Muscles

In the lateral abdominal wall, from the thorax to the pelvis, run four abdominal muscles which are arranged in two pairs each crossing at right angles (strapping) in the directions of the fibers. One pair represents the straight strapping with the *M. rectus abdominis* running lengthwise, and the *M. transversus* running across. The other pair represents the oblique strapping with the *M. obliquus abdominis externus* which has a backward-downward fiber direction and the *M. abdominis internus* which runs forward and downward.

The ***M. rectus abdominis***, the **straight abdominal muscle**, runs in the form of a flat muscle lengthwise next to the midline and is connected from the sternum to the crest of the pubic bone by the tough tendinous mass of the *Linea alba* with the same muscle on the other side.

Origin: Outer surface of the sternum and the cartilage of the ribs in the area of the 4th to 8th (9th) rib, therefore, essentially, on the cartilages of the supporting ribs.

Insertion: With a strong end-tendon which merges with the abdominal tendon of the *M. obliquus abdominis externus* on the pubic bone.

Branches: 1. *Tendo femoralis recti*, a tendon cord of the thickness of a small finger, which attaches itself to the *Caput femoris*.
2. *Tractus symphysicus recti*, the prepubic tendon, which runs down to the pelvic symphysis.

Function: The *M. rectus abdominis* is suspended between the sternum and the pubic bone like a hammock; the weight of the intestines rests upon it. Approximately ten tendinous transverse strips are inlaid in its long fleshy body. Although the muscle fibers run in the lengthwise direction of the entire muscle, the lifting height is not diminished, but the work strength is increased tenfold.

The ***M. transversus costarum***, the **transverse muscle of the ribs**, can be seen as an extension. It prolongs the *Rectus abdominis* in the form of a flat, weak band of muscle, joined together by a mutual tendinous sheet, and ascends from the cartilage of the 4th rib to the end of the 1st rib. It holds the first four ribs together and, thus, also strengthens the point of origin of the *M. scalenus* to a small degree.

The ***M. transversus abdominis***, the **transverse muscle of the abdomen**, has its muscle body above and its flat tendon below in the lateral ventral abdominal wall.

Origin: With a short aponeurosis on the transverse spinous processes of the lumbar vertebrae on the inside of the cartilages of the last 12 to 13 ribs.

Insertion: With its broad tendon from the xiphoid cartilage until a hand's-width in front of the crest of the pubic bone on the *Linea alba*, meeting head-on with the other side.
The transverse muscle of the abdomen has no attachment on the pelvis.

Function: Suspensory apparatus for the abdomen.

The ***M. obliquus abdominis internus***, the **oblique internal muscle of the abdomen**, has its muscle belly above and behind, on the coxal tuberosity, and its broad tendon with fiber direction to the front and downward in the lateral and ventral abdominal wall.

Origin: Coxal tuberosity and *Fascia iliaca*.

Insertion: By means of muscle on the last rib and on the inner surface of the cartilage of the 18th to 15th rib; with its broad abdominal tendon, it fuses in the *Linea alba* with that of the other side.

Function: It suspends the thorax on the coxal tuberosity and serves as a suspensory apparatus for the abdomen.

The ***M. obliquus abdominis externus***, the **oblique external muscle of the abdomen**, has its muscle belly at the front and above, namely externally on the costal wall, and its broad tendon with fiber direction to the back and downward in the ventral and lateral abdominal wall right up to the coxal tuberosity. One should distinguish an abdominal and pelvic tendon on the oblique external muscle of the abdomen.

Origin: On the outer surface of the ribs from the 4th (5th) to the 18th in a slightly ventrally bent serrated line from the point of the elbow to the loins.

Insertion: 1. Its abdominal tendon is fused in the *Linea alba* with its counterpart from the other side, therefore, firmly anchored at the back on the crest of the pubic bone.

2. Its pelvic tendon goes to the coxal tuberosity, to the *Tracto inguinalis* and *Tendo praepubicus*.

3. Its *Lamina femoralis*, which extends from the pelvic tendon right over to the inner surface of the femur, merges into the *Fascia medialis femoris*.The abdominal skin muscle also meets the inner surface of the femur together with the fascia.

Function: This muscle joins the sternum to the pelvis and, as all other abdominal muscles, serves as a suspensory apparatus for the abdomen. It also works together with the abdominal skin muscle in moving the hind limbs forward. Furthermore, all abdominal muscles constitute the abdominal press, which play a role in breathing out; it is responsible for the bursts of exhaled air as the horse snorts.

See Chapter 2 on the role of the abdominal muscles in stabilising the torso, Chapter 6 on their role as muscles of movement.

The ***M. cutaneus maximus***, the **abdominal skin muscle**, is the main section of the large skin muscle of the torso, on the lateral surfaces of the chest and abdomen, which, as it lies subcutaneously, closely joins with the *Latissimus dorsi* and also with the *M. pectoralis profundis*. Toward the front, it continues as the skin muscle of the shoulder onto the shoulder-upper arm area, but it also connects with the *Crista tubercoli minores* of the humerus by means of accretion on the *M. teres major*. Toward the back, narrowing to a point, it radiates into the back of the stifle and allows its aponeurosis to extend onto the inner surface of the femur, where it blends together with the femur sheet of the oblique external abdominal muscle into the *Fascia medialis femoris*. This connection from the front to the hind leg determines the tension of the muscle and the skin in relation to the positions of the legs and to the movement (Chapter 7).

Selected Bibliography

1. **Becher.** Reflections on the natural method of training. German Sankt Georg sports magazine (38th year of publication), No. 21, 22, 24, 26 (1937/1938).
2. **Bittner, H.** Article on the mechanics of the thoracic vertebrae of the horse. Archive of scientific and practical animal medicine, 56, page 236 (1927).
3. **Borcherdt, W.** Studies of the jumping movement of the horse. Inaugural dissertation, Bern (1912).
4. **Born and Möller.** Handbook of Horse Care. 9th edition, published by Parey, Berlin (1928).
5. **Busow, R.** Speed and Stamina. Illustrated review of thoroughbred breeding and racing, H.1, page 38 (1936).
6. **Camus.** Article on the study of movement of the horse, the neck muscles in combination with the front limbs. Military veterinary manual, Volume 19, No. 4. Page 561-570. Ref.: Veterinary journal, Volume 48, page 158 (1936).
7. How mechanical laws of balance, movement, and bridles and bits. The Cavalry Journal Ref.: Veterinary journal, 24, 142 (1912).
8. **Disselhorst, R.** How to judge the Horse. Published by Parey, Berlin (1923).
9. **Dreyhausen, G. von.** Lectures on the science of equitation. Published by the Cavalry School, Hannover (1931).
10. **As above.** The fundamental concepts of the art of riding. Published by the race- and campagne riders' association, Vienna (1936).
11. **Duerst, U.** Judging the horse. Published by Enke, Stuttgart (1922).
12. **Ellenberger-Baum.** Comparative anatomy of domesticated animals. 17th edition, published by Springer, Berlin (1932).
13. **Ellenberger-Scheunert.** Comparative physiology of domesticated animals. 3rd edition, published by Parey, Berlin (1925).
14. **Gmelin, W.** The external structures of the horse. Published by Schickhardt and Ebner, Stuttgart (1925).
15. **Haase, F.** The relationship between the movement of the horse and the influence of the rider. Analysis of the gaits of the horse. Published by the Cavalry School, Hannover (1932).
16. **Haugk von.** The training of the young military horse in the snaffle bit. Published by Mittler and Son, Berlin 1929.

17. **As above.** The movement and training of the horse. German Riding Jounrals, 1937, H. 26-28, 1938, H. 4-8.

18. **H. Dv. 12 German Cavalry Manual of Horsemanship,** Xenophon Press, 2014.

19. **Heydebreck, von.** Military and civilian riding instructors and riders. Published by Mittler and Son, Berlin (1938).

20. **As above.** The working horse and its training. Published by Mittler and Son, Berlin (1935).

21. **Hilgendorff.** "The horse works through the poll" is based on its anatomy, posture, its mechanics and how it is ridden. Veterinary Journal, 36, 238 (1924).

22. **As above.** The anatomy of the horse is the basis of its performance and dressage. Veterinary Journal, 45, 353 (1933).

23. **Kadletz, M.** The changing shape of the muscles of the hindquarters of the horse during movement. Viennese veterinary monthly journal 1926, page 187.

24. **As above.** On the physiological circulation and the static function of the shoulder extremity; as well as an attempt to explain so-called "Struppiertheit" and "Fuchteln". Weekly Munich veterinary journal 83, 433 (1932).

25. Reflections on the cavalry with special emphasis on the training of young horses. Our horses, Stuttgart 1897.

26. **Klingemann.** The bars of the horse's mouth from the point of view of a veterinarian and rider. Veterinary Journal 43, 124 (1931).

27. **Koch.** Constriction in the throat latch. Veterinary Journal, 45, 138 (1933).

28. **Knebusch.** Tension in the horse and solutions. Our horses, Stuttgart (1911).

29. **Köhler.** To what extent problems connected with how the horse is ridden result in false diagnoses and how these mistakes can be avoided? Veterinary Journal 49, 49-62 and 81-102 (1937).

30. **Kronacher, C. and Ogrizek, A.** The conformation of the horse in relation to the angle of the limbs and the length of the stride. Breeders' Journal, Series B, Volume, 23, page 184 (1931).

31. **Krüger, W.** The functional reinforcement of the fascia in large domesticated animals. Extra volume of the Anatomical Journal 72, 159 (1931).

32. **Linkenbach,** Exercises to encourage understanding and trust between horse and rider. Published by the Cavalry School, Hannover (1932).

33. **Löwe, K.** Observations of the German thoroughbred. Veterinary Journal, H. 2, (1938).

34. **Magnus, R. and De Kleijn, A.** Posture and position of the limbs of mammals. Excerpt from the handbook of normal and pathological physiology, distributed by Bethe, Bergmann, Embler, Ellinger. 15th volume, 1st part. Published by Springer, Berlin 1930.

35. **As above.** Posture, balance, and movement in mammals. Ibidem.

36. **Meller.** Anatomical reasons for riding young horses with the neck extended from the point of view of the rider. Veterinary Journal., 44, 426 (1932).

37. **M. H. B.** Working the young military horse from July until the beginning of October. Our horses, Stuttgart (1902).

38. **Monteton, O. von.** Purchasing young horses for military work and their training. Our horses, Stuttgart (1899).

39. **Natzmer, O. von.** Riding with pleasure. 3rd edition. The German Publishing Union, Stuttgart (1937).

40. **Paulli, S. and Sörenson, E.** The fascia of the horse. Special publication of the Royal Veterinary School of Medicine, Copenhagen (1930).

41. **Rau, G.** Judging the warmblood. 2nd edition, published by Parey, Berlin (1936).

42. **As above.** The cavalry manual: the war horse. Published by Schickhardt and Ebner, Stuttgart (1936).

43. **As above.** The international art of riding at the 1936 Olympic Games. Published by Sankt Georg, Berlin.

44. **Sanden, V.** The influence of dressage, exercise, and obedience training on the military horse. Our horses, Stuttgart (1898).

45. **As above.** Various concepts on the training of the riding horse. Our horses, Stuttgart (1901).

46. **Schauder, W.** Anatomical and metric studies on the muscles of the shoulder extremity of the horse. Scientific and practical archive of veterinary medicine, 47, H. 3, page 237 (1921).

47. **As above.** The fetal "development of the tendons" of the horse. Archive of microscopic anatomy and mechanics of development, 102, H. 1/3 (1924).

48. **Schilling.** What does "natural balance" and "balance under the rider" of the horse mean? Which muscles are used to balance the horse under the rider and how do they function? Veterinary Journal 43, 156 (1931).

49. **Siems, H.** Riding and obedience training. Published by the Reher Commission Co., Berlin (1933).

50. **Schmaltz, R.** The anatomy of the horse. 2nd edition, published by Schoetz, Berlin 1928.

51. **Simon.** Static and mechanical function of the equine skeleton. Veterinary Journal 34, 1 (1922).

52. **As above.** The balance of the horse in static mode and under saddle. Cavalry School, Hannover (1924/25).

53. As above. Anatomical observations on articles in the "Sankt Georg" magazine on how the function of the back of a correctly moving horse functions and on collection. Veterinary Journal, 38th year of publication, H. 4, page 97 (1926).

54. Spohr. Injury at speed of racing and riding horses. Our horses, Stuttgart (1897).

55. As above. The logic of the art of riding. On the rider's aids in riding and dressage relative to mechanical function of the anatomy of the horse. Our horses, Stuttgart (1903).

56. As above. Part II. Elementary dressage based on aids appropriate to the mechanical function of the horse. Our horses, Stuttgart (1904).

57. As above. The condition of our military horses, how to achieve and maintain it. Our horses, Stuttgart (1912).

58. Steinbrecht-Plinzner. Gymnasium of the Horse. Xenophon 1994.

59. Srubelt. On the importance of the *lacertus fibrosus* and *tendo femor tarseus* for standing and movement of the horse. Archive for scientific and practical veterinary medicine, 57, H. 6, page 577 (1928).

60. Thörner, W. Physiological sport studies of trained dogs. Research and advances 13, 12 (1937). Ref. D.T.W. 30, page 482 (1937).

61. Walter, K. The movement sequences of the free limbs of the horse in walk, trot, and canter. Inaugural dissertation, Berlin (1925).

62. Wegener, H. Studies of top horses from the jumping and dressage yards of the Cavalry School Hannover. Published by Schaper, Hannover (1934).

63. Wenger, F. Article on the anatomy, static, and mechanical functions of the spine of the horse. Inaugural dissertation, Bern (1915).

64. Zietschmann, O. Movement. Excerpt from Stang-Wirth, animal medicine and breeding. Published by Urban and Schwarzenberg, Berlin-Vienna (1926-1937).

Xenophon Press Library

www.XenophonPress.com
Xenophon Press is dedicated to the preservation
of classical equestrian literature.
We bring both new and old works to
English-speaking riders.

30 Years with Master Nuno Oliveira, Henriquet 2011
A Journey Through the Horse's Body, Fritz 2012
A Rider's Survival from Tyranny, de Kunffy 2012
Another Horsemanship, Racinet 1994
Austrian Art of Riding, Poscharnigg 2015
Broken or Beautiful: The Struggle of Modern Dressage, Barbier/Conrod 2020
Classic Show Jumping: the de Nemethy Method, de Nemethy 2016
Classical Dressage with Anja Beran, Beran 2021
Collection or Contortion: Anatomy and Biomechanics of Positioning and Bending, Gerd Heuschmann, Doctor of Veterinary Medicine, 2024
Divide and Conquer Book 1, Lemaire de Ruffieu 2016
Divide and Conquer Book 2, Lemaire de Ruffieu 2017
Dressage for the 21st Century, Belasik 2001
Dressage in the French Tradition, Diogo de Bragança 2011
Dressage Principles and Techniques: A Blueprint for the Serious Rider, Tavora 2018
Dressage Principles Illuminated, Expanded Edition, de Kunffy 2021
École de Cavalerie Part II, Robichon de la Guérinière 2015
Elements of Dressage, von Ziegner 2022
Equestrian Art: The Collected Early Writings (1951-1956), Nuno Oliveira 2022
Equestrian Art: The Collected Later Works, Nuno Oliveira 2022
Equine Osteopathy: What the Horses Have Told Me, Giniaux 2014
Essence of High School Method of Captian Raabe, Decarpentry 2023
Federico Grisone's "The Rules of Riding," Grisone/Tobey 2023
Fragments from the Writings of Max Ritter von Weyrother, Fane 2017
François Baucher: The Man and His Method, Baucher/Nelson 2013

French Equitation: a Baucherist in America, 1922 & Hand-book for Horsewomen, Bussigny 2023

General Chamberlin: America's Equestrian Genius, Matha 2020

Great Horsewomen of the 19th Century in the Circus, Nelson 2015

Gymnastic Exercises for Horses Volume II, Eleanor Russell 2013

H. Dv. 12 German Cavalry Manual of Horsemanship, Reinhold 2014

Handbook of Jumping Essentials, Lemaire de Ruffieu 2015

Handbook of Riding Essentials, Lemaire de Ruffieu 2015

Healing Hands, Giniaux, DVM 1998

Horse Training: Outdoors and High School, Beudant 2014

Horsemanship & Horsemastership Volume 1, US Cavalry 2021

Horsemanship Training Films 3 DVD set, US Cavalry 2021

I, Siglavy, Asay 2018

Journey Through the Horse's Body, Dr. Christina Fritz 2022

Learning to Ride, Santini 2016

Legacy of Master Nuno Oliveira, Millham 2013

Lessons in Lightness: Expanded Edition, Mark Russell 2019

Mark of Clover, Barczy Kelly, 2022

Methodical Dressage of the Riding Horse, Faverot de Kerbrech 2010

Military Equitation or, A Method of Breaking Horses, and Teaching Soldiers to Ride, Pembroke, and *A Treatise on Military Equitation*, Tyndale 2018

My Horses Have Something to Say, de Wispelaere 2021

Principles of Dressage and Equitation, a.k.a. Breaking and Riding, Fillis 2017

Racinet Explains Baucher, Racinet 1997

Releasing the Jaw, Poll, and Neck DVD, Mark Russell 2021

Riding and Schooling Horses, Chamberlin 2020

Riding by Torchlight, Cord 2019

Riding in Rhyme, Davies 2021

Seat, Gaits & Reactions, de Sévy, 2023

Schooling Exercises In-Hand, Hilberger 2009

Science and Art of Riding in Lightness, Stodulka 2015

Sketches of the Equestrian Art, Barbier/Sauvat 2022

The Art of Riding a Horse, D'Eisenberg 2015

The Art of Traditional Dressage, Volume 1 DVD, de Kunffy 2013

The Chamberlin Reader, Chamberlin/Matha, 2020

The de Nemethy Method: A training seminar, 8 DVD set, de Nemethy 2019

The Ethics and Passions of Dressage Expanded Edition, de Kunffy 2013

The Forward Impulse, Santini 2016

The Gymnasium of the Horse, Steinbrecht 2018

The Horses, a novel, Walker 2015

The Italian Tradition of Equestrian Art, Tomassini 2014

The Maneige Royal, de Pluvinel 2010, 2015

The New Method of Dressing Horses a.k.a. A General System of Horsemanship, Cavendish 2020

The Portuguese School of Equestrian Art, de Oliveira/da Costa 2012

The Quest for Lightness in Equitation and Equestrian Questions, Nelson/L'Hotte 2021

The Rider forms the Horse, Udo Bürger & Otto Zietzschmann, 2024

The Rules of Riding Gli Ordini di Cavalcare, Grisone/Tobey 2023

The Spanish Riding School & Piaffe and Passage, Decarpentry 2013

The Spanish Riding School: The Miracle of the White Horse DVD, US Lipizzan Association 2021

To Amaze the People with Pleasure and Delight, Walker 2015

Total Horsemanship, Racinet 1999

Training Hunters, Jumpers, and Hacks, Chamberlin 2019

Training Your Foal, Ettl 2022

Training with Master Nuno Oliveira, 2 DVD set, Eleanor Russell 2016

Truth in the Teaching of Master Nuno Oliveira, Eleanor Russell 2015

Wisdom of Master Nuno Oliveira, de Coux 2012

Printed in the USA
CPSIA information can be obtained
at www.ICGtesting.com
CBHW040327030324
4764CB00001B/2

9 781948 717564